love lay down beside me and we wept

with very best wishes
Helen

HMT
2025

ALSO BY HELEN MURRAY TAYLOR

The Backstreets of Purgatory

love lay down beside me and we wept

Helen Murray Taylor

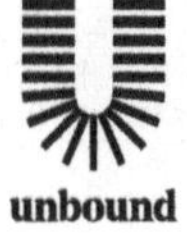

First published in 2025

Unbound
An imprint of Boundless Publishing Group
c/o Crimea House New Road, Great Tew, Chipping Norton, England, OX7 4AQ
www.unbound.com

Typeset by Jouve (UK), Milton Keynes

A CIP record for this book is available from the British Library

ISBN 978-1-80018-348-3 (hardback)
ISBN 978-1-80018-349-0 (ebook)

Printed in Great Britain by Clays Ltd, Elcograf S.p.A

1 3 5 7 9 8 6 4 2

For my family and friends. With love and gratitude.

Contents

Glasgow

I

How do you write a memoir when your memory has gone up in flames? When what remains of the past smoulders so faintly that you can barely make it out? But then it flares up and blinds you, so you can't tell what's real and what's not?

Fortunately, I kept notes.

2

When I was twenty-eight, I bought myself a violet linen minidress from the sale in Jigsaw, Covent Garden. Ten years later it was the dress I was wearing when I killed myself.

The dress was plain in shape, cut on the bias, with capped sleeves and a wide neckline that almost hung off my shoulders. The linen cloth was criss-crossed with diamonds of fine stripes in dark purple. In its simplicity, it was little short of a classic. You could say a little short, full stop. When I bought it, we'd been living down south for two years but I had not adapted. The humid summers in central London still managed to get their sticky fingers into me. The city aggravated an already precarious state of affairs, a steady anxiety-sweating that threatened to burst into a torrent under the most minimal provocation and that even industrial-strength antiperspirant was incapable of damming. I wore my new dress once in the height of summer and then, mortified by the deluge which appeared under my armpits and at the base of my spine and turned the violet black, I never wore it again.

That was, at least, until many years later when I discovered that the lithium I was taking miraculously stopped my anxiety-sweating. The drug dried my mouth and made my tongue stick to my teeth when I spoke. It set off tremors in my hands and in my legs, and it made my head shake of its own accord. It made me unable to walk in a straight line and it turned my writing to a microscopic scrawl that could only be read with a magnifying glass.

But it opened up a plethora of wardrobe opportunities.

For ten years the Jigsaw dress lay screwed up at the bottom of the wardrobe until I decided, for no particular reason, to resurrect it that morning. Given my decision-making capacity at that time, that in itself was an act of unusual resolve. Despite being bombarded daily with well-meaning advice along the lines of small steps to be taken one after another, the reality was that I was barely capable of choosing which foot to put forward first, never mind which shoes to wear while doing it. It is odd that I should have chosen that particular day to select an untried, untested, almost entirely new (give or take a decade or so) outfit. But that is what I did.

The smell at the back of our wardrobe reminds me of my gran's house, a nostalgic smell that had persuaded me to persuade Mark that our first flat was definitely worth buying (*I feel at home here*), a smell I associated with oak floorboards, threadbare rugs from distant lands and antique furniture, but which I later came to realise was actually woodworm, damp and stale fags. And so, on that morning, clutching my find, I resurfaced from the wardrobe depths and assessed the crinkled linen. As expected, it had a vague whiff of raw oak and neglect, but the smell was not unpleasant. When I held the dress up by its drooping shoulders it looked several sizes too big for me, but that didn't worry me either. After the weight I had lost, it would show off my collarbones to their razor-sharp best. I tried it on. Peering over the knobbles of my shoulders, I admired first one side and then the other in the wardrobe mirror. My hair hung limply down my back. My legs dangled below the hem like pieces of loose thread. I smiled at myself, pleasantly impressed by what was reflected, blinded no doubt by the excitement of the big day. During the wilderness years, I was delighted to remark, the dress had not gone out of fashion. Mainly, of course, because it had never been in.

Impressed though I was, I couldn't stay all day admiring myself. There were things to be getting on with.

In London, the dress had been a summer dress to be worn (the once) with bare legs and sandals, but this was Glasgow and it was already September. Summer was drawing its last asthmatic breaths. I pulled on black leggings and shoved my feet into a pair of double-tongued, low-rise Converse.

A few hours later, wearing that very dress and the rest, I was to be found in the resus room of A&E at the Western Infirmary, half comatose and fading fast, while some poor house officer tried and failed to get a line in me.

Of course, it is facile to blame the dress. But the facts are irrefutable. Whichever way you look at it, there is no way it would have been possible for me to pass the afternoon in my garden swallowing pills and swigging back gin on 2 September in the thirty-eighth year of my life wearing that particular Jigsaw dress if, ten years earlier, I had left the shop empty-handed.

So, fuck it. I'm blaming the dress.

★

You don't have to be a brain surgeon to work out that I didn't actually die. But the deceit here is not that I survived. The deceit is that I write flippantly, as if it is something to laugh about. It isn't funny. Nothing about suicide is funny. Not for the person who completes or doesn't. Not for those entangled in it or those forsaken by it. And not for those left asking if they did enough.

I crashed several times that night. I've asked Mark for details but he is too traumatised to remember more than impressions. Cardiac arrest. Ventricular fibrillation. Asystole. Clinically dead but not until they call it.

I don't know who saved me. I don't know who pumped my heart or cleared my airway. I don't know who masked me and turned on the oxygen. I don't know who cut through my dress and stuck on the defibrillator pads, who charged the machine and shocked my heart. I don't know who found an open vein for the IV, who injected the adrenaline, or who intubated me and attached me to a ventilator. I don't know who stuck the central line into my neck, who threaded the arterial line through my femoral artery, who titrated the drugs to bolster my failing heart, to stop my blood pressure plummeting and my kidneys from failing. I don't know who treated my seizures and my pulmonary oedema. I don't know who monitored my pulse, my oxygen levels, my brainwaves, my fluid balance. I don't know who and I don't know how many.

But I do know what it is like to skirt the edges of death.

There was no tunnel. No white light.

There was no rush of memories. No ciné reel of my life.

There were no angels. No spirits. No precipices. No falls.

There wasn't a shower of bliss or a jolt of terror. I didn't float above the drama watching the panic to resuscitate me. It wasn't any of the things you hear. Any of the things you might expect. Any of the things you might hope.

I'll tell you what it was.

It was a big, fat, fucking, gold-star anticlimax.

It was exactly . . .

Nothing.

3

Mark doesn't want to be in this book, but I can't write this story without him. He was there from the beginning. Right in the middle of this tangle of love and death and madness.

Love came for me in a canteen salad bar on my first day of university. In all my wildest imaginings (and trust me, they were plentiful), I would never have believed that a plateful of pasta salad, tomatoes, lettuce, grated carrot, tuna mayonnaise and honey-roast ham (our anatomy-class-induced aversion to cooked flesh was yet to manifest itself), not to mention a curried rice salad, a Waldorf knock-off, coronation chicken (the seventies were long gone but their legacy lived on in institutional cooking), cucumber slices and a beetroot affair (malt vinegar included), plus a bread roll and a packet of crisps (salt and more vinegar) could totally give me the hots, while I simultaneously questioned whether someone so skinny could actually put that amount away.

I had already spotted Mark around campus in Freshers' Week and I wanted to be his friend. He had long, dark, curly hair that hung over his face, and clothes that, in my amateur but enthusiastic opinion, walked the trendy side of goth (as if such a thing existed) – black trench coat, stick-leg black trousers and a shirt that would have been the envy of his Purple Princeliness. I'd seen him wafting around the Student Union in a manner that, given his hair completely obscured his sightline, was irrefutable proof of his familiarity with the place. At gigs, he stood at the back, hunched over a chin-stroking plastic glass of Southern Comfort and lemonade, while the band played and the mosh pit flailed. Moments later, he'd hit Dance Floor Central, feet and elbows a blur. It was a little surprising that he could dance at all, given how pointy his black patent-leather winklepickers were, but he managed without restraint. I found him – his attire, his moves, his beverage – radically cool. What I could see of his face behind his hair (limited for the most part to the flash of grinning teeth) was, my heart assured me, to die for. All of this heightened by his hand-waving speech which, had I been near enough to hear, I would have discovered was accompanied by the jangle of a wristful of cheap bangles. I was smitten. But my awe kept me circling at the outskirts of his field while he remained entirely unaware of my existence, laying waste to the paradigm that opposites attract.

If I mention it now, he teases me. 'I wasn't cool,' he says. 'You just didn't know any better.' Back then I was just a girl from the sticks. I feign outrage.

I met him properly a week later. It was our first official day of university and we were in the queue to matriculate.

'Hi.'

'Hi,' I said back, shyness and manners preventing me

from explaining that he was in the wrong queue. That this one was for medics and dentists.

'I'm doing medicine,' he said. The first of a lifetime of occasions he would read my mind.

We registered for our course, signed where we had to sign, and picked up our student cards. On the way out, he hooked up with a bunch of people he knew from school and dragged me along with them for lunch. In the canteen, Mark and his schoolfriends piled ahead of me in the queue. I trailed behind. For the sake of appearances, I ordered one item from the salad bar while my insides churned over whether I could justify the unplanned spending. A furtive glance reassured me that no one had remarked on my profligacy.

Mark, on the other hand, worked his way along the salad bar ahead of me picking the aforementioned selection of items. He didn't realise they were charged per spoonful and not per plateful. The cashier rang up the till.

'Four pounds forty-six,' she said (or some other extortionate amount). I flinched on his behalf. Those were the days when you could still withdraw £5 notes from an ATM, an amount that, if I was careful and rationed my lager habit, could stretch to an entire week.

'Oh,' he said. 'Can I put something back?'

She stared at him, letting the unbending polyester stripes of her tabard answer for her. Behind him, the clatter of crockery, the pressure of plywood trays sliding along the stainless-steel runners hassled him. Ahead, the clang of cutlery, the scrape of chairs, the babble of the lunchtime crowd pulled him onwards. He shrugged and paid up.

At this pragmatic and unflustered display, my stomach shot somewhere into my chest cavity and my skin turned inside out. I couldn't actually believe what I had witnessed. I gawped in admiration. My brain shrank a little away from my skull and swelled again on the rebound as I handed over my carefully counted forty pence for my single scoopful. Had I fallen in love or was I getting a migraine?

4

How did it happen? How did I go from love to the edges of death?

5

When I was seven years old, one of my sisters made a breathless announcement.

'Everyone!! There's a bald man walking up the path.'

We all rushed to the window to check. Sure enough, it was true. There he was, winding up the garden path between the pansies in the rockery and the twisted willow tree that the cat used as a scratching post, and he was smiling and waving to us. This bald man's presence would prove an interesting diversion to the normal Saturday routine of supermarket shopping and meeting Dad afterwards in the Legion for a pint (or a bitter lemon or Pepsi and, if we played our cards right, a packet of smoky bacon). He was, it transpired, my dad's older brother, who had come to pay us a visit. Over the course of the weekend, we discovered that his baldness was not his only distinctive attribute. He was also a kidney-transplant surgeon. Once I'd scoured my Junior Pears Encyclopaedia to discover what a kidney was, I found the idea of transplanting them pretty stupendous. There and then, I decided to follow in his footsteps. When I grew up, I declared to anyone who was willing to listen, I was going to be a doctor. Through childhood and adolescence to young adulthood, it remained an unfaltering conviction.

The first two years of medical school did nothing to dent this conviction. They were two years of glittering happiness with Mark beside me as my best friend. The academic work didn't really present me with a challenge. A rigorous study habit and neatly written lecture notes balanced the raucous laughter, the messing about in the back row of lecture theatres and the speedily completed labs. I sailed through. But Mark's notes were illegible and his study erratic and he didn't make it. He was devastated. When I moved on to third year without him, I was lost. In the hospital, habit made me search for him to sit beside at coffee break or lunch. I had other friends, but his absence filled the empty seats.

As pre-clinical students, we'd been desperate to see real live patients, but clinical work was not what I had hoped. An inexact science and fallible bodies that wilfully ignored the gospel of our textbooks meant that I was always going to find it tricky. But there was more to it than that. There was something about me that didn't fit. It wasn't just the skirts home-sewn from brightly patterned offcuts from the bargain bin in Remnant Kings, skirts that skimmed the top of my Doc Marten boots, or the oversized cardigans with nibble holes at the wrists. My clothes were clearly some kind of statement, though I couldn't tell you what. The rest I couldn't put my finger on.

In the staff room, six medical students nervously wait to go into battle, the lads among us fidgeting and sparking static in their shop-new Next suits. We leap to our feet when the professor strides in. A brief pep talk and he sweeps off again, leaving us under the command of the registrar. In vowels as crisp as his starched white coat, the registrar introduces himself. He is tall, clean shaven, officer material, and wears his name badge on his breast pocket like a medal. He strides the length of the line to assess the standard of his troops. When he reaches me, he stops. 'Are you here to work or to party?'

'Sorry?'

An arm gesture and a sneer about my get-up. Asks me what I was thinking when I got dressed that morning and accuses me of having no respect for the patients. I'm mortified. It hadn't occurred to me that my clothes would be considered disrespectful.

'White coats,' he says. 'The lot of you.'

Quick-smart we put them on and troop out onto the ward behind him. After a brief lesson on the fundamentals of clinical examination on some obliging patients, it is our turn. We march past a couple of beds and stop at one in the second bay. The registrar swishes the curtain closed and we fight through the opening to assemble around the bed.

'You.' The registrar is pointing at me. 'Neurological examination of the lower limbs.' Five other medical students ready and willing, and he trains his sights on the one who is already mortally wounded.

I push through the others to reach the bedside. The registrar is on the opposite side. The patient is a frail woman in her late seventies. She is propped up on several pillows. Her thin hair is sticking out at all angles and her teeth are in a plastic beaker on the bedside cabinet.

'Is that OK?' I ask. 'If I examine your legs?'

After a few moments of flustering to work out how to lower the back rest of the bed, I finally succeed. I am leaning over her while she lies flat. My white coat is not buttoned. 'I do like your dress, dear,' she gums. 'Very cheerful.'

She giggles when I tell her I can make her one. The registrar is scowling. I ought to get on with it. I pull down the bedcovers and begin the examination, mentally ticking off what we have been taught. First: observe. I carefully study her legs for any differences, for signs of muscle wasting, for other abnormalities. Nothing obvious. Second: muscle tone. I rest my hands on her twiglet thighs and roll her legs from side to side. Under the crisp sheet, the waterproof mattress squeaks. I put my hand behind her knees and bend her legs, straighten them. Her muscles don't seem particularly rigid or unusually slack. Maybe the left is slightly stiffer than the right. Hard to say. I check that she's OK. She is nodding along in encouragement. Move on. Third: strength. I get her to lift one leg off the bed, then the other, and then again while I push down on them. Her left leg appears weaker than her right. Should I report my findings? I hesitate. Hear a tut. Pistol-crack sharp. I flinch. Have I made a mistake already? Am I taking too long? I must be taking too long. Should I test all the other muscle groups in detail or will that wind the registrar up further? I whizz through the rest of the examination and then pause to glance at him, fully expecting him to bawl me out for whatever cardinal student crime I have committed. He glowers at me. *Carry on.*

Next step: reflexes. I start with her feet. Without warning, I scrape the pointed handle of my reflex hammer along the outside edge of her left sole. Her foot jerks away from me.

'Sorry,' I whisper.

'It isn't your fault, dear,' she whispers back.

'Can I try again?'

She nods. *Ready.*

This time her big toe briefly flexes upwards. Or does it? I can't be 100 per cent sure. I ask if she minds if I repeat it once more. I hear a salvo. *Tut tut tut tut.* Ignore him, I tell myself. Concentrate while under fire. Yes, definitely upward flexion. Babinski reflex positive. A sign of neurological damage. Babinski positive plus left-sided weakness equals stroke. I snatch another peek at the registrar. Shall I move on or is he expecting a summary? 'Why do you keep stopping?' he says. 'What's wrong with you? It's like you are constantly seeking approval. It's pathetic.'

A collective gasp from the rest of the group. I admit I am taken aback by the attack. But the thing is, he is right on both counts. I *am* seeking approval and it *is* pathetic. A futile attempt to pre-empt the criticism that I sensed from the start. 'It's because you keep tutting,' I go. 'You are putting me off.' I giggle conspiratorially with the patient.

Mistake. The crime of insubordination. He barks his scathing opinion of my attitude. I'm stunned. How has he got me so wrong? Can't he tell that I am a girl with top-of-the-class syndrome and a pathological desire to please? I stutter a few words in self-defence but he doesn't want to hear them. He tells me to get out of his sight, to go, to leave the ward before he really loses his temper.

'You're joking, right?' We have regressed from the army back to school. Apparently, I am a misbehaving teenager to be sent out of the class.

'Do I look like I'm joking?' He certainly does not look like he is joking. He is flexing his fingers as if he would gladly strangle me. 'Get off my ward.'

I laugh. This is mad. It is our first day. Who gets chucked out on their first day? I can't actually believe this is happening.

'Go!' He is shouting now. Drops of spittle strafing the bedclothes.

Suddenly, it isn't a laughing matter. I can't even pretend to find it funny. I turn to the patient and pull the bed-covers back up over her. I am shaking. She clutches the covers up to her heart. 'I'm really sorry,' I tell her. 'You shouldn't have had to witness this.'

'It's all right, dear. It's not your fault.'

With as much dignity as I can muster (which isn't very much), I leave the ward. The rest of the group are gawping in my wake. I seem to have forgotten how to walk normally. My hips sway unnaturally. My knees jerk strangely with each step. My feet are twitching to scarper but I am determined not to run. As soon as I reach the staff room, I tear off my white coat, grab my bag and flee to the library, where the rustle of academic journals and the slip-clunk of the photocopier will muffle my gulps and tears of rage.

Although our paths crossed no more than a couple of times afterwards, reiterations of that confrontation echoed through every clinical encounter that followed. It was easy to blame the registrar, but the real enemy was my own terror of being less than perfect. If I was asked to examine someone and describe her heart murmur, the rustle of her nightdress against the barrel of my stethoscope whispered contempt at my ineptness. In the wheeze of asthmatic lungs was a sneer that even I couldn't miss. The ketotic breath of diabetes blew scorn over me with its sweet poison. I came to dread my morning walk from Buchanan Street Underground, up Cathedral Street, past the old maternity hospital on Rotten Row and on to Castle Street, where the blackened stone of the Royal Infirmary loomed before me, and the sense of history and the stories of the patients who had passed through its high-ceilinged wards were scratched into the bricks. The high-flown spires of the Gothic cathedral next door and the sepulchral skyline of the Necropolis behind only added to my sense of foreboding.

On the ward, there was no room for error. When our tutors quizzed us, if I wasn't absolutely certain of an answer – and generally even when I was – I kept my mouth shut. I was so terrified of putting a foot wrong that I barely put a foot anywhere except into my black-and-white stripy tights in the hope that, somehow, they would do the talking for me. My bedside manner was a mixture of tortured silence peppered with explosions of strident learning.

In the staff room next to the ward, I would check my pen torch for batteries, shove my stethoscope and notebook in my pocket, and thread the long handle of my reflex hammer through a buttonhole of my white coat, where it would inevitably bash my legs when I walked, and thus hindered and weighed down by the tools of my trade and my fear of messing up, I'd join my fellow students on the ward to demonstrate my rudimentary skills to our clinical tutor and whoever else, real or imagined, was there to cringe at the spectacle.

6

It wasn't all bad. My crazy flatmates kept me sane with nights of laughter verging on hysteria. Mark was my keystone. The one that stopped everything collapsing around me. On Saturday lunchtimes he bought New York hoagies from the sandwich shop two along from the pharmacy where he had a part-time job, and we ate them in my room out of the paper bags rather than risk dismantling the tower of dirty dishes in the kitchen sink. Weekend nights we'd cadge free passes to the Sub Club or splash out on tickets for gigs at the Barrowlands. On Sundays I'd scrounge a roast lunch at his mum's to supplement my diet of Dad-grown tatties and tinned tomato soup. And if there were weekends where my studying was up to date or I didn't have a netball match, we went on trips to Edinburgh or home to see my family and schoolfriends. Kipping on the floor in the bed recess in my pals' kitchen, our breath mingling with the after-smell of veg chilli. Midnight, walking along a frosty beach, frozen hand in frozen hand and shoved deep into the pocket of Mark's coat, gazing up at the infinite night sky, convinced that we were hallucinating the shooting stars. Waiting outside the bar where he worked and spotting him in the distance, bouncing along, late for his shift, and then inside, huddled in a corner reading a book while he poured pints. Hearing the creak of the huge wooden door of the Reading Room and the echo of footsteps on the parquet and glancing up from my books in the hope that it was him. There were times when life came between us but, somehow, we always found our way back to one another.

Meanwhile, at uni, I was breezing through the academic subjects, sweating through the clinical practice. As finals approached, I was too preoccupied to notice the disparity. But by the time I graduated, the enormity of what was ahead began to bother me. Was I actually ready to go onto the ward as a real-life doctor? As 1 August approached, stress began sucking out of my brain every morsel of medical knowledge that I had been accumulating over the previous five years. On the day I collected my junior house officer name badge and my pager, I felt so ill-prepared and ignorant, it was as if I had never attended a class.

The first time I was in charge of the cardiac-arrest pager, I found myself in a state of wide-eyed, bristling panic. A friend gave me some advice that belied the five years of training that we had both had.

'When you hear the arrest beeps,' he said, 'run.' The faster the better, he assured me. 'It makes it look like you know what you're doing.'

And I could run with the best of them.

7

It was medieval times. Barbaric times. We worked a one in three. That is to say, every third night we worked all night. Not instead of our normal eight-to-six day or whatever we were doing, but as well as. We had a routine. The night after a night on call was the night for sleeping. The night after that was the night for going out. There were many blurred two or three o'clock in the mornings where we'd find ourselves debating whether to carry on drinking and clubbing or to call it a night. The question we were really asking was whether sleep or alcohol was a better way to silence the doubts. At the end of the evening, my voice echoing around the back courts of the tenement flats before I staggered my way home, the usual protest refrain: 'Guys, I'm on call tomorrow.'

If you were in a good team or on a good ward, there was solidarity in the misery. If you were still roaming the wards at 5 a.m., some kind soul would usually make you tea and toast. After an all-nighter, your workmates might take your pager so you could slip away early. But the fatigue was killing, and it wasn't long before I found myself envying the patients in a coma, or sometimes even the patients who were dead, and I was ready to sacrifice anything for a sleep that peaceful.

The strain was beginning to show, in the raw patches of eczema at the angle of my nose, in my eyes that were puffy and bloodshot, in my hair that had lost its shine. The mirror didn't lie and neither did my patients. On the surgical ward, one of the patients on my blood round was a young lad whose leg had been amputated after he'd injected temazepam into his femoral artery. Normally my interactions with him were a spark of relief. He was upbeat and funny, and spent his time racing around the ward on his crutches, bothering the nursing staff and entertaining us with his banter. But that day I wasn't in the mood. We were the receiving ward for the day, expecting emergency referrals from A&E or directly from GPs. I was on call, with a long and very busy day and night before me. It wasn't even 9 a.m., and my bleep was already hassling me non-stop.

To get ahead, the previous evening I had prepared all the sample tubes for the day's bloods, placed them with syringes, antiseptic wipes and balls of cotton wool into cardboard trays, which I had piled high, ready to be done in the morning before the early ward round. That morning, I had already laughed at the Dracula joke for the gazillionth time but nonetheless appeared to have made little impact on the teetering mountain of trays. The lad with the amputation was next on my list. Every junior doctor knew that IV drug users were a nightmare to bleed. If they were in for surgery, it was a pretty safe bet to assume they had a long-term habit. Which in turn meant veins that had suffered with use. I was too busy to mess about. Didn't have time to be held up by a patient with non-existent veins. Anticipating difficulties, I fastened the smallest-calibre needle onto the head of the syringe, loosened the clip from the tourniquet and did a quick survey of his forearms. His skin was patterned with scars of old drug tracks. No chance of an open vein. How was I going to drain even a few measly millilitres? Twanging the tourniquet between my fingers, I scanned his hands, his good ankle, the top of his foot in search of a vein that wouldn't collapse at the sight of the needle, blinded by the list of tasks scrolling inside my head: results to chase up, X-rays to order, drugs to prescribe, fluids to write up, pager to answer.

'Hand it over, doc.'

'What?'

'Hand it over. I'm better at this than you.' He nabbed the tourniquet and fastened it around his thigh. I passed him the needle and syringe and watched with relief as he skilfully extracted blood from a cobweb of a vein at the ankle of his remaining leg. Once he was done, he handed back the syringe and said, 'You look wrecked, by the way.'

'Charming,' I said, attempting to laugh, but I couldn't disguise the fact that I was on the edge of tears. Today I couldn't take insults, jokey or not.

'What car do you drive, doc?'

'A turquoise Citroën AX,' I answered, taking the syringe off him and squirting blood into the tubes. 'Why?' I gave him an exaggerated glower of fake suspicion as I bagged the samples and the corresponding forms. Was he going to take the piss out of my car too?

Turns out he was looking out for me.

'Give us the registration and I'll make sure it isn't nicked.'

Newcastle

8

For my senior house officer job, for reasons that are beyond me, I applied for a medical rotation in a district hospital in a small town not far from Newcastle. At the interview I dazzled and cracked jokes. I don't know what was up with me. A few weeks later I packed up my Glasgow flat into a couple of cardboard boxes. On the drive down south, I played my car stereo at full volume and shouted along to ward off my tears, wishing I was brave enough to turn the car around and go back home to Mark. Halfway there, I stopped at a service station on the A1 to fill up with petrol and go for a pee. I was in the loo when a bloke shoved the door open, almost taking it off its hinges.

'You're supposed to lock the fucking door,' he shouted at me in disgust.

'I did,' I said, but my protest was little more than a whisper. For the rest of the journey, I cried tears of humiliation and grief and prescient homesickness.

My hospital accommodation was a room above the mortuary. I imagined that steeped in the threadbare carpet and the dust-laden curtains was the stench of death. To alleviate the gloom, I decorated the room with belongings I had brought from home and from my trips abroad for my student electives: brightly coloured batiks from The Gambia, a woven bed-throw from India, a balsa-wood model of a Gothic building that Mark had given me the first Christmas I had known him. I had my record player, my vinyl collection, my Penguin Modern Classics. There was even Ted, straw-stuffed and ageing, who slept on my pillow with the agreement that if anyone popped in, he wouldn't complain if I shoved him in my bedside cabinet in an effort to maintain the illusion that I was a grown-up with a proper job. But however many souvenirs of happiness I displayed, none of them, not my music, not my books, not even my sweet, old teddy bear, brought me any comfort.

The ward I was assigned was without a permanent consultant. There were locums who stayed a week or two. Between locum consultants, I was nominally in charge. A typical ward round would go something like this.

8.30 a.m. Ward 19. I am wheeling the trolley of case notes up the ward. The steering is more temperamental than your average supermarket cart. A staff nurse is multitasking between me and three patients.

'How are you today, Mrs Jackson?' I ask, hauling the latest volume of her epic medical history from the trolley. The case notes open with a thud and I scan the most recent entries.

'Fine, pet. I'm waiting to see the doctor.' She is sitting next to her bed. Her face is partly hidden by the wings of the high-backed chair. I move around the trolley to take a better look at her. Her static pink nightie tones with the light-blue vinyl of the chair. The nightie, the chair cover,

Mrs Jackson: they all look washed out. I suspect she may be anaemic.

'I'm the doctor today, Mrs Jackson,' I say, just as the staff nurse arrives. Glances are exchanged. I take Mrs Jackson's wrist. Under my fingertips is the stutter of her pulse. Atrial fibrillation. I take a quick glance at her blood-pressure chart. 'Can I have a wee listen to your heart?'

'Of course, you can, dear.' I dive in to listen. Her voice booms through my stethoscope as she chatters to the staff nurse. 'Did she say that she's the doctor? She's very young. Do you think she sat her A levels when she was twelve?'

When I resurface, I pull the stethoscope out of my ears and scribble in her case notes. I order bloods, an ECG, a chest X-ray and a review of her medication, all of which will be up to me to organise.

Before we wheel the trolley off to the next patient, out of badness I tell Mrs Jackson that I didn't sit A levels. The shock on her face makes her look like a fish. A fish about to have a heart attack. 'Scotland. We do different exams,' I explain hastily, so as not to leave her terrified that her medical care is under the charge of an unqualified child. Even if that is how I feel most of the time.

Mark did his best to understand the pressure of the job, but it was asking the impossible. He couldn't really understand. Nobody could, not my non-medic friends, not my family, not the nurses we worked with (the patients were much more aware of the hours we put in than the staff). Because unless you had done it yourself, unless you had trawled the wards for close to sixty hours on the trot during an entire weekend on call so that by the end of Monday you couldn't string two words together, unless you had eaten nothing but yellow disc Quality Streets for breakfast, lunch and dinner, or, every time you tried to make a dash to the toilet, been accosted to write up a pharmacy order or a fluid chart or do a quick once-over of Mr Jones because he was looking a bit peaky, or been woken from your snatched ten-minute snooze in the drugs cupboard by the insistence of your pager, unless you had doled out IV antibiotics with as much sparkle as an ailing zombie, it was impossible to comprehend the sheer annihilation of that bone-breaking, mind-dislocating fatigue.

On the few weekends that I had free, I drove weary-eyed up to Glasgow. There in the pub where Mark worked, to the background clamour of fruit machines and whisky-fuelled debates, I'd drink my pint at the bar and flirt with the manager, and if I played my cards right, he would do me the favour of letting me pretend to be staff – empty the ashtrays and sweep the beer-sticky floor after closing – and let me stay for the lock-in. For which I was pathetically grateful.

9

To escape the stench of death, I moved out from the mortuary room to a terraced house in Newcastle. It had coughing gas heaters, prickly carpet tiles and a leak behind the shower that dripped through the kitchen ceiling, but it was, nevertheless, an improvement. I had two housemates who dried their underpants in the microwave and who could occasionally extract a laugh from me with their antics but who couldn't stop me bringing my patients home. Not literally, obviously, because there wasn't a spare room and I wouldn't have subjected to them to my housemates' debatable hygiene practices. All the same, it wasn't long before my home had become a squat for the septic, the maimed, the terminally ill. Patients shook me awake from sleep, crashed my breakfast, blasted me with the cold shower when I fell asleep in the bath. They weren't genuine hallucinations, because I saw them and heard them inside my head, not outside. Still, they floated from the pages of the journals I was using to study for my post-grad exams, they appeared at the bottom of a beer bottle at the end of a long night, they jumped out at me from my wardrobe first thing in the morning. It was a horror show. There were patients nursing the stumps of limbs that had been incorrectly amputated. Patients with blood smeared around their mouths and spewed into kidney bowls from upper GI bleeds I had missed. Patients unconscious with subdural haematomas I'd put down to being pissed. Rashes from mismatched transfusions. Infections from injections into Hickman lines that I hadn't kept completely sterile. Patients accusing me of putting symptoms down to a minor case of gout when I'd missed a major case of gangrene. Dying of a heart attack I'd dismissed as indigestion. Hundreds of them, queuing up to show me the contents of their sputum pots, their ECG traces, their ultrasound scans, constantly questioning whether I had made the correct diagnosis, ordered the appropriate tests, prescribed the correct drugs. I was growing so terrified of missing a critical diagnosis that I was in danger of becoming the type of doctor likely to treat an ingrowing toenail with a below-knee amputation, a graze with a skin graft, a headache with a brain transplant. Just to be safe.

It wasn't sustainable. Soon, I was barely eating, barely sleeping. I regularly woke at 4 a.m. and couldn't get back over. To rid myself of the bitter taste that permanently washed my mouth, I got into the habit of cleaning my teeth five or six times a day, minimum. I was afflicted with a constant headache that I put down to my eyesight getting worse from being forever stuck in my books. The PMT that had always had me jumpy and teary each month tipped me over into weeping buckets. All these signs. All these signs that were so obvious. All these signs that I refused to acknowledge because there was no way on earth that I was admitting to anyone, especially not to myself, that the only job I had ever wanted to do was not working out.

In May of that year, I went on holiday to Fuerteventura

with my parents and my younger sister. The wind howled and sandblasted my sunburnt skin, and at the peak of the dormant volcano, the bushes moved of their own accord. It made me question my grip on reality, but it transpired we'd cycled into the middle of a training exercise for the French Foreign Legion. The others laughed at the absurdity, but I couldn't find anything funny.

I was walking a precipice.

I would have slipped eventually, I'm sure, even if the wind hadn't flung me off the cliff.

10

Slow-motion horror. A motorcyclist blown off the flyover. An image imprinted in my brain. I slam on the brakes. Ahead of me, a Transit van skids. In vain. No time to swerve. Direct hit. The motorbike crashes to the ground ahead of its rider. The rider thumps off the windscreen of the van and straight under its wheels. It trundles over him with a sickening thud that I can't have heard but clearly remember. The van driver is frozen in his seat, his hands gripping the steering wheel. In a trance, I put on my hazards and step into the nightmare, knowing already that what is about to happen will scar me for ever.

I dash over to the injured motorcyclist. A young lad, no more than a teenager. His injuries are horrific. Crush injuries to his chest and abdomen. All four limbs twisted at unnatural angles. Possible broken neck or spine. Blood pouring from the angles of his lips. He is still conscious. Groaning and gurgling on the blood that has filled his mouth.

Behind me, other drivers have stopped and are getting out of their cars.

'Does anyone know first aid?' someone says. A reluctant volunteer steps forward.

'It's OK,' I say to the crowd. 'I'm a doctor.' Not that I

reckon I am better qualified to help. I say it to take the burden from the others, aware consciously or subconsciously that the outcome is inevitable.

I kneel down beside the boy. Loosen the strap of his helmet. Panicking, the first-aider shouts at me not to remove it.

'I'm not going to,' I say. I'm pissed off. 'I'm trying to clear his airway.'

I put my finger in the boy's mouth to scoop out some of the blood. A futile effort. He needs suction to clear his airway. If I was at work, in ICU, I would have all the equipment that was needed. The boy's jaw is in pieces. The other bones in his face are shattered. A quick survey of his status shows that almost every bone in his body is crushed. Any intervention I make risks putting him in danger, but if I do nothing, he is going to die. I make a half-hearted attempt to turn him to the recovery position, but he is too damaged. It feels like he will fall apart. Traffic is crawling past, some drivers getting twitchy because they will be late for work, because they haven't seen what is unfolding next to them. I yell for someone to stop the cars until they find someone with a mobile phone. A rare thing in those days. 'Call nine-nine-nine,' I shout. 'We need an ambulance, police. We need help.' I tell the boy he is going to be OK. He knows I am lying. The veins in his hands have collapsed. His skin is pale. Cold. His body is shutting down. Internal bleeding. No external bleeding that I can stem. He needs fluids, a transfusion. I have to get a line in him while I still can. But I don't have a cannula. I don't carry supplies in my car. Someone offers a blanket and fetches it from their boot. I take it to keep him warm but the gesture isn't for him. As I wrap it around him, I shift his body. He gargles in pain. I flinch in apology and take his hand. Feel the unnatural slip of the bones in his wrist. I tell him again that he is going to be OK, that the ambulance is on its way. At least this time, my words hold some truth.

It is minutes before the paramedics arrive but time has congealed around us. When they arrive, they take over. Under their revolving blue light, they swing into action. Even with their full kit, they struggle to get a line in him. I volunteer to have a go but they won't let me. I am getting in the way. They splint the boy's head and neck, stretcher him into the ambulance. The sirens blare and he is gone.

I get back into my car and turn off the hazards. It is way after 9 a.m. and I am going to be late for work. A flash of misplaced stress makes me angry for the delay. I have patients to attend to in ICU. I have a consultant waiting for me to show up. But when I go to drive off, I am stuck. I sit with my hand on the ignition key, churning over the scene. Horror sweeps over me and I'm questioning whether I was about to take off his helmet, what might have happened if I had. Had I missed a source of bleeding that I could have stopped? Did I harm him when I tried to turn him to the recovery position? What if his neck was broken and I had exacerbated it? What if had I been too quick to tell myself that his injuries were beyond help? If – when – he dies, will I have to take some of the blame? And at the same time, inside I am yelling at myself that it is academic, that I couldn't have done anything to save him, that nobody could have, that it isn't my fault. It isn't my fault. It isn't. Getting my version of the story ready to convince others as I try to convince myself. I am desperate to get back to the carefully controlled environment of the hospital, where there is a specific protocol for resuscitation, where there is at least the semblance of control of external factors. I start the engine. Drive slowly past the police taking a statement from the van driver. Drive past the wreckage of the motorbike. The motorway is strewn with tangled metal and shattered glass from the windscreen of the van. I see the discarded blanket. I see splashes of blood where the boy had been lying. And then I notice them, thrown across the carriageway. A pack of tuna sandwiches wrapped in clingfilm, packed by the boy's mum that morning, and planned for the lunch he was meant to have. When he was still alive.

Death, as a junior doctor, was part of the fabric of the day. Emotional detachment was a prerequisite. We coped with bad jokes and bravado. The formalities helped too. Expected or unexpected, there were procedures to deal with it, protocols to follow, families to inform, death certificates to complete, post-mortems to arrange. In the real world, there were no such formalities to protect us.

At work later that day I heard on the news that the boy had died. The registrar asked if I wanted to go home, but I stayed to finish my shift. My next weekend off I fled to my childhood home. In desperation, I sat for hours on the sand dunes at the beach, watching the rising tide and the beckoning sea. I didn't have the courage to answer its call. When darkness fell, the black waves crashed against the moon-grey sand, and the night sky was icy clear. Finally, bone-stiff and desolate, I turned and made my way home.

11

The accident hollowed me out. It would revisit me in all its forms, in versions where I did better, in versions where I did worse, and came to represent the sum of my worth as a doctor – and as a human being – however well I was doing on the ward. Superficially, I was a high-flier, with my consultants happy to have me on their team and the first lot of post-grad exams successfully under my belt. But there was nothing inside where any confidence in my ability should have been. It would be my undoing.

When I was alone, I wept. From the day of the accident and every day that followed. I wept on my weekend drives to Glasgow. And on the long drive back down the road. In the locked bathroom of my house when the housemates were home. On my trawls around the city in the evenings, assessing the jumping quality of the bridges over the train line. Every night in bed before the nightmares. At the end of the phone to Mark, my friends, my family. At the hospital before my day started, I'd stop off in my on-call room and cry screwed-eyes-ugly, full-flow-snotty, trembly lipped, stuttered-breath tears. And then I would compose myself and step onto the ward.

Until the day came when I couldn't do it any more.

It was my sister who heard it. The desperation in my unspoken words at the other end of the telephone. She begged me to come home. I went off sick. I never went back.

12

Post-traumatic stress disorder as a diagnosis I could just about deal with, but depression didn't fit with my image of myself. However much the psychologists and counsellors stressed that it wasn't my fault, that I wasn't coping because I was unwell, that I needed time to recover, their reassurances were meaningless.

I had been exposed as the thing I feared most. A failure. My identity had been plastered together from exam passes, certificates, qualifications. But there was no substance to it. I was a construct of a person, a papier-mâché model, and I was collapsing in on myself.

For months I dashed between towns – between my house in Newcastle, Mark's Glasgow flat and my parents' place up north – never staying long enough for anyone to poke their fingers through my paper-thin shell.

'I'm not sure this is good for you, this peripatetic lifestyle,' my counsellor said.

And there's me, open-mouthed that he would blatantly admit he found my lifestyle very pathetic. I protested but I was inclined to agree with him.

*

I slept late, read and watched bad telly. I swallowed anti-depressants and hours of counselling. The drugs dissipated the worst of the depression, and the counselling conned me, temporarily at least, into believing that the world wouldn't end if I messed up a bit. Slowly the tears dried up. I ventured out to buy the daily paper for the crossword, I cooked the odd meal, I completed a claim on my medical sickness insurance before my sick pay fizzled out. When eventually I dared to show my face to friends, someone said that I didn't look depressed. It was true. The break had given me the chance to catch up on sleep and regroup. In many ways, I looked no different from my usual self. But each time I considered returning to clinical medicine, fear, panic and a storm of tears smashed over me and left me battered and utterly deflated.

It wasn't going to work. I wasn't mentally or physically capable of getting myself back on the ward. Medicine was all I had ever wanted to do. It was the only version of the future that I had ever considered. The only version where I felt my life had any worth. I couldn't see what else would give it shape and meaning. But I had to find something. It would be criminal to waste the education and opportunities that I had been given. And apart from anything else, I had to find some way to pay the bills. The insurance company weren't going to pay out for ever.

The obvious choice was medical research. My student electives to The Gambia and India had sparked in me a fascination for tropical medicine and parasitology that I was keen to explore further. Research would suit my academic inclinations without the responsibility of having someone's life in my hands. But at the same time, I felt guilty. Research seemed to lack the vocation, the altruism, that I considered central to being a physician and which was the varnish that I thought had given me value. Plus, I would have to get more qualifications – an M.Sc., a Ph.D. – and the idea of going back to university felt completely self-indulgent. Study for the pleasure of it.

Once I was accepted on to a course at the London School of Hygiene and Tropical Medicine, I spent a lot of time aggressively defending my choice to others and to myself. The remaining months I spent dossing in Mark's flat waiting for the academic year to start and one-finger typing letters for his Ph.D. application. I wasn't going to repeat my mistake of moving away without him.

Mark was offered a Ph.D. in Oxford with a decent bursary. I had a scholarship to cover my fees and sold my car to bolster a year with no income. We piled our possessions into the back of a rented van and set off for new beginnings, with the leaves of Mark's fig plant tickling my ears in the driving seat. *You are now leaving Glasgow*, the sign said. *Have a safe journey*. Bumping along in the van down the M74, we passed Gretna Green and it felt like we were eloping in the wrong direction. Another sign, *Welcome to England*, and before long we were driving through the Cumbrian hills, where I caught glimpses of my early childhood: over Shap, where Dad's car had broken down when we were kids on a trip to visit my gran; the heart-shaped forest growing on the hillside with its myth of the grief-stricken widower – which I wanted to believe, and not just that, hemmed in by a V of dry-stone walls, it had grown that way by chance; Ingleton Quarry; the arches of the Ribblehead Viaduct; the mudflats of Morecambe Bay and a fleeting sight of my old home town in the distance.

As we drove south, the landscape flattened and the motorway got more and more jammed. We stopped for lunch at Sandbach services. It was packed. Once we had queued for our food, I sat opposite Mark at a ring-marked table eating my Filet-O-Fish and searching his face for signs of regret. From time to time I still ask him whether I bullied or blackmailed him into coming with me. He claims it was neither, but I suspect it was both.

Oxford and London

13

My map-reading skills were not all they should have been. It turned out London and Oxford were actually a very expensive season ticket apart. After some emergency financial planning, I threw myself into study, doing most of my work on the train on the daily commute back home. I was hooked. It was a pleasure to use my brain-power to do thinking, not worrying. Life was easy. Our college flat looked out over the River Cherwell, with its moorhens, spring cygnets and summer punts. There were tennis courts in the grounds, sheds for the bikes we used to go everywhere, and a hushed modern library to study in. Whatever spare time I had, I spent playing netball for the local town club. For the first time in ages, I was physically and mentally fit.

Late spring in that first year. The warm weather was coming but there was still a sharp edge to the evening air. Mark and I were walking back to our college flat from Raoul's cocktail bar after several of their notorious multi-measure Long Island iced teas when a woman passed us with a baby in a buggy.

'I want one of those,' I said. My second niece had just been born. I was in love with her and her older sister.

'Even if you're not married?' Mark said.

'You what?' I said, flabbergasted and about to launch into a tirade.

'No, no, no, I didn't mean it the way it came out,' he said in a panic before I could go off on one. 'I meant to say, "Will you marry me?"' As proposals went, it was outstanding in its clumsiness. But I didn't care. I was delirious.

We bought a bottle of fizzy wine from the corner shop and drank it in the college gardens, and that weekend we bought the funkiest engagement ring ever from an art gallery in Oxford. A hot-pink tourmaline. It looks like a sucked Jelly Tot. It is beautiful.

It rained the day we got married. August in the north-east of Scotland, and the record-breaking heatwave broke, and the haar engulfed the bay and the crumbling castle on the headland. The tiny sandstone church and its graveyard were engulfed by the mist and it felt like a world apart. Mark and his best man, my soon-to-be brother-in-law, sneaked behind the war memorial to calm their nerves with swigs from a hip flask while the guests milled between the gravestones, drunk on the heady scent of rapeseed and sea air. My sisters were bridesmaids, my brother the chauffeur in my dad's car, and my tiny nieces the flower girls. The electric organ wobbled on its spindly legs to a tune that no one recognised (including me, despite having chosen it), the minister stopped our appalling singing mid-verse as an affront to religious decency, and my toddler nieces lay in the aisle and flashed their fancy knickers. The ramifications of a dwindling congregation and a minister nearing retirement were soon to take their toll. We were the last couple to be married there.

Later, we ate and danced and laughed in my mum and dad's garden. The haar pushed up against the flaps of the marquee and made the ceilidh sweat. The guests loosened their ties and kicked off their heels. The photos show us glowing with happiness, Mark in a hired kilt and all the trimmings, me in a fine-pleated Beverly Lister dress with a full-length veil and three-inch heels that made me taller than him. We were twenty-eight. As darkness fell, the rain spattered off the canvas and the earth sighed in petrichor and mud.

Sometimes I think that the rain was an omen. It nourished the earth like our friends and family nourished our marriage.

14

The Oxford days were bathed in light. Warm tones of honey and flax that glowed off the ancient stone suffused in centuries of history and learning. The elitism and the sense of entitlement that often resounded around the quadrangles in plummy vowels were intimidating, but together Mark and I were proud outsiders. After my M.Sc., I started a Ph.D. at the research institute at the John Radcliffe. All year round we cycled to work. Past the frost-glittered lawns and primrose carpets of University Parks. Up Jack Straw's Lane, where the bluebells peeped between the roots of oak trees or midges caught our throats. Into Headington and towards the hospital, wheels clicking over tarmac sticky with summer heat or splashing through autumn puddles.

In the lab I began with the basic practical skills of molecular biology – extracting DNA and RNA, amplifying specific fragments by PCR, running gels, Southern blots, Northern blots, gene sequencing – before I moved on to more complicated techniques for the analysis of the parasite genes I was interested in. Everything about the lab thrilled me. The equipment, the chemicals, the specialised kits. The calamine scent of phenol, the nail-varnish-remover tang of acetone, the Marmite smell of the yeast extract in the broth for culturing bacteria. Powdered detergents that triggered a coughing fit even if you were wearing a mask. The black-pudding aroma of stale blood from the incubators for the malaria parasites.

My project was to analyse the genes that were responsible for the constantly varying proteins that the malaria parasite exported to the surface of the infected human red blood cell as part of its strategy to escape our natural immune response. I started on parasites that had been adapted for growing in the lab and later spent a couple of months in Kenya working on wild strains. The hours I worked were up to me, but I freely gave up evenings and weekends to finish an experiment or feed the parasites. Apart from the Sunday when Mark phoned me in the lab to say that he had just met David Bowie in the local newsagent, I never resented the hours. Given a choice, I would have done more. I couldn't have been happier.

Every Tuesday lunchtime, four of us from the lab, the self-styled junior squash league, took our amateur ball skills to the squash court. What we lacked in skill – we were easily outclassed by the expert players – we made up for in expended calories. We'd compete until we could barely stand, weighed down by the litres of sweat clinging to our t-shirts, legs weak from dehydration and from killing ourselves laughing at comedy mishits.

Oddly, though, there were signs that things weren't quite as bright as I was making out. I had developed a hand tremor that dictated how high to fill my coffee mug without the risk of sloshing it, and the troublesome anxiety-sweating that determined which clothes I could and couldn't wear. It was weird. I didn't feel anxious or nervous. It's true that the first time I had to give a presentation, I was terrified and in awe of the intelligence and reputations gathered in the seminar room, but I pulled it off and afterwards was buzzing with the high of success. Subconsciously, I put the tremor and the sweating down to being a bit hyper because I was always on the go in the lab or at netball training and weekend matches. But there was more to it than that.

Almost without my realising, it was beginning to sink in what a tricky career academic science was. It wasn't just that your experiments might fail, that your hypotheses may prove to have no merit, that you could invest years of work to find yourself at a dead end. The problem was how much of it was outside of your control. Just because you worked hard didn't guarantee results. Just because you had a great idea didn't mean it would pay off. For every success, there was an unquantifiable element of luck. And then there was the funding, short-term contracts, the precarious future. I can't tell you how many brilliant scientists dropped out of academia for jobs with long-term security or pay that would support a family. Meanwhile, out the corner of my eye, I watched my medic friends progressing with their careers. I refused to admit to envy. I was doing something that I loved. I don't know if I ever consciously formulated the fear, but it was there in the background. I had already failed once. I couldn't fail again.

15

Ambitious, driven, competitive. That was me. Introverted, anxious, self-critical. Also me.

After our Ph.D.s, Mark and I moved to London, me to start a research post at the National Institute for Medical Research and Mark to start a proper job with prospects and security. For the first time in four years, we were not solely reliant on scientist wages or student grants. We bought a flat in Hornsey, passing itself off as the more desirable Crouch End, and, once we'd installed a damp course and condemned the gas cooker, lifted the carpets and sanded the floorboards, we painted over the flowery wallpaper and furnished it with finds from the junk shop at the corner of Priory Park and Middle Lane. The cat came from a notice in the newsagent two streets away. Flea-ridden and with an appetite for chewing electric cables, she immediately dug her needle-sharp claws into our hearts and didn't let go.

The first London summer was concrete-heat, hay fever and the smell of the Underground. My parents visited on their way home from a holiday in France with my two eldest nieces, by then aged eight and five. Mark and I took the girls swimming at the lido in Crouch End where, like the responsible pretend parents that we were, we slathered them in sunblock, squeezed armbands over chubby arms, and splashed around in the cold water with ducks and seagulls swimming alongside. After we had jumped in approximately 72 times, after I had rescued them 46 times from Mark the Shark, after we had been It at least 311 times, I was standing in the shallow end with the little one in my arms. She was uncharacteristically quiet. I took my swimming goggles off and had a good look at her. She was totally blue. Our first attempt at parenting and we had given the poor creature hypothermia. After an emergency towel-dry and change, and panicky auntie cuddles to transfer some body heat, we made them both promise not to tell their mother or their grandparents.

Later that afternoon we all went to the park to fly the kites their grandparents had bought them on holiday. The photos show the kites – pirate galleons – in splendour against a clear blue sky and the two girls with smiles beaming brighter than the sun. That evening we went to Wagamama for dinner and instilled in them both a lifelong weakness for chicken katsu curry. Maybe something we got right as pretend parents.

'I wish they were nearer,' I said. We had waved them off early in the morning, the girls and my mum with their hands out of the car windows and me standing in the middle of the road on tiptoes until Dad's car disappeared out of the end of our street and towards their journey home. Now Mark and I were out for a drink in All Bar One, having a glass of Sauvignon Blanc that by the end of the night would turn into most of a bottle. We were sitting at a rickety wooden table that wobbled no matter how many beer mats we slipped under its feet, and unconsciously mirroring each other wiping condensation off the outside of our wine glasses. A bit teary, I tried to describe the sensation when they slipped their little hands into mine and how their soft skin against mine made my heart skip a beat, but my words didn't do justice to the emotion of it. Trying to describe love was like trying to stroke Schrödinger's cat.

'Maybe we should think about having one of our own,' Mark said. We both sort of giggled. Since his dodgy marriage proposal, the subject of babies had barely arisen. For nearly five years we had been too skint and the future too undecided to consider the idea. It seemed ridiculously grown-up, something that we wanted but that was always, would always be, in the future. It wasn't as if we were particularly young, though. We were both thirty-two. If we meant it, if we were serious about having a family, we should probably get on with it. Leave it much longer and it could get tricky. Obstetrics classes at medical school had taught me that a first-time mother just a couple of years older than me would be described in the extremely flattering and not-at-all-misogynistic term of 'elderly primigravida'. I didn't feel old, but the medical profession obviously thought otherwise. The term a not-so-subtle hint that we should get going asap, perhaps. But ambition had to have its tuppence. Was this a good time? What about my research? Could I afford to take time out? If I wanted to make a name for myself, should I get more papers under my belt? I was a late starter, after all. Was it possible to be a mother and a successful scientist? There were few women in academic science who hadn't made some sacrifices either to their career prospects or to their prospects of having a family. The nature of the job ensured that it was often either/or – career or children – however talented or however ambitious you were. I wanted both. I wasn't the first and I wouldn't be the last. But what if I couldn't make it work?

'If anyone can do it, Helen,' Mark said, 'you can.'

I squeezed his hand.

So that was it. We were proper adults. We were going to have kids. Hilarious.

16

The babies didn't come. We had fun trying but after a while it was just trying.

There were constant phone calls from friends with news. News I always dreaded. I'd clutch the receiver and sit on the back step watching the cat stalk butterflies in the garden, and do my best not to let my voice betray my rictus grin as I asked for the due date and how they were doing. And I'd gush with congratulations and squeak how happy I was for them when, in reality, I was insanely and toxically jealous.

After a year, we went for tests.

17

Before I went under, they made me sign a consent form to allow them to slice me open for a full laparotomy. In case the micro-slits of a laparoscopy weren't big enough to extract the cysts. 'But that never happens,' the gynaecologist assured me.

I woke up disorientated and attached to a drip, with a 15-centimetre incision smiling above my pubis and the worst abdominal pain I can remember. I peeked under the covers. My hospital gown had ridden up around my waist and the wound dressing was stained with seepage. They had, however, hooked me up to a morphine pump, so it wasn't all bad.

The nurse told me the ovarian cysts were bigger than expected. The doctor would be round after theatre to give me more details. Nothing she said gave me particular cause for concern. But that might have been the morphine.

For the rest of the day, I dozed in my bed next to the nursing station with my drip hand resting on the starched sheet that covered me, or lay staring up at the cathedral ceiling, marvelling at the bore of the heating pipes, all the while listening to the reassuring hum and click of the morphine pump, which was just audible above the clatter of the ward. Over the course of the day, the saline drip was replaced several times. I was nothing if not well-hydrated. The trauma to my pelvis during the surgery, however, had caused my bladder to protest. It filled and filled until I looked six months pregnant. The irony wasn't lost on me. Eventually, one of the nurses had a moment and sat me on the commode.

I couldn't pee. The pain of my bursting bladder was untouched by the morphine. I sat there straining and crying. My bladder was about to rupture. I foresaw collapse, panic buttons, emergency surgery. I had to get help. Before it exploded. Before it was too late. Right on cue, the curtains swished open, revealing me in all my indignity to the whole ward. The surgeon preened and commenced to show me the photos of the huge cysts he had removed from my ovaries.

'This big one is an endometrial cyst,' he explained with pride. It was glistening and purple and resembled a mutilated jellyfish.

'Jesus Christ,' I said. 'Can I have some privacy?'

He left, shirty with me for not appreciating his stellar work, and didn't bother to pull the curtains back around.

The diagnosis of endometriosis caught me unawares. I should have guessed. Years of horrendous period pain and fatigue, cysts and infertility. It didn't take a genius. And clearly, I was no genius.

A nurse inserted a catheter and the urine flooded from my traumatised bladder. I topped myself up with morphine and wept. They moved me to a side room so I wouldn't disturb the other patients.

The following day, a different gynaecologist came by. He might have been a registrar.

'We're going to put you on danazol,' he said.

'No way,' I said. Danazol is a synthetic testosterone. It brings on a chemical menopause.

'It is the best treatment,' he said.

'On what fucking planet? I'm trying to get pregnant.' I was practically yelling. Hadn't he read my notes? On another day, I might have swung for him, but this was today and I was afraid of bursting my stitches. I settled for moral superiority. 'I wouldn't take it anyway because of the side-effects.'

'What side-effects?' he asked, put out.

'Oh, I don't know,' I said. 'Let me think. Maybe the ones that give you a masculine jawline and make you grow a beard?'

He washed his hands before he left the room. I was discharged without follow-up.

18

We had four rounds of intrauterine insemination, or IUI for short, on the NHS. IUI is no longer available as a treatment on the NHS for couples in our position because the data have shown that it is no more successful than doing nothing. We didn't know that at the time, although a gynaecologist friend hinted as much, but at least it made us feel like we were making an effort. My memory of that summer is endless mornings in obstetrics outpatients at the Whittington Hospital, with the sun streaming through the streaks on the windows while I waited for scans or to have the procedure, surrounded by pregnant women and new mothers and posters about breastfeeding and childhood vaccinations and my billowing resentment. And afterwards, I'd slip back to work, maybe hide out in the fluorescent microscope suite or skip lunch and coffee breaks, whatever it took to avoid having to come up with an excuse for my comings and goings.

After four attempts at IUI we had used up our allocation. Each one had failed before I even had the chance to do a pregnancy test. I had got what I deserved. Punished for the arrogance of thinking I could have it all.

*

In the lab, we occasionally ran short of blood supplies to feed the malaria parasites. If a phone call to the transfusion service at Colindale revealed there were no out-of-date packs that we could use, we had to improvise, or the parasite cultures would crash and weeks of work would be wasted.

'Can you bleed me, H?' one of my co-workers asked one afternoon. Qualified medics only were permitted to wield a needle and syringe.

'Sure, no problem,' I said.

She assembled the equipment while I washed my hands. It had been more than three years since I had taken anyone's blood, but I had had so much practice in the past, been so proficient, I didn't anticipate it causing me any real problem.

'Ready?' I asked.

'Yes. Are you?'

I fastened the tourniquet, slipped the butterfly cannula into her vein, drew off two fat syringes of 50 millilitres, and squirted them into the orange-capped centrifuge tubes ready with anticoagulant.

'Gosh, H,' she said when I was done. 'I've never seen anyone's hands shake that much before.'

19

The first appointment for IVF had none of the physical indignities of the ones which were to come, but it was difficult in other ways. In the waiting room, we whispered and avoided eye contact with other couples. Before we met the consultant, we were given leaflets to read, leaflets which boasted of their state-of-the-art facilities, their pioneering treatments, their unsurpassed success rates. It wasn't until much later that I understood their interpretation of 'success' would not be the same as mine. At reception, overlooked by a pastel collage of baby photos and glowing new parents, we worked through a folder which described in detail what was to come. We filled out forms. Consented to HIV tests. Shrugged off the option of counselling. The receptionist deftly moved on to outline the costs. Assessment, tests, monitoring, drugs, scans, egg extraction, fertilisation, implantation, anaesthetic. Somewhere in there was the price of the fresh flowers in the waiting room and the subscription to *Harper's Bazaar*. Her practised eye noted the beads of sweat on my forehead as we signed the consent forms.

We left the clinic dazed. On Marylebone High Street, we stood for a moment – traffic crawling alongside and bags of luxury shopping jostling us on the pavement – debating whether we should both go back to work. Mark asked me if I wanted a coffee.

'A drink,' I said. 'I need a drink.'

The heavily disguised, curtained entrance of the Sanderson Hotel made a pretence at modesty but, in reality, it was designed to keep us out. Neither of us could tell which was the window and which was the door, so there we were, feeling foolish, both of us chivvying the other to test it out. Somewhere in a back room the security men watching the CCTV must have been pissing themselves laughing. Just as we were about to risk humiliation, a shiny-haired, suited, moneyed crowd swished through the entrance and we followed them inside before the doors closed ranks.

At the bar, we ordered cocktails, started a tab. Rum and fresh raspberries, a martini with lavender pollen. We perched on bar stools, silently holding hands while the drinks were mixed. When they were ready, I left mine sitting on its paper coaster and leaned forward to drink it through a straw, clasping the neck of the glass with both hands to control the wild shakes that were now a constant affliction.

We drank until the suffocating lilies and the plush leather sofa that had swallowed us up in the clinic waiting room became nothing more than a bad memory.

'Are we doing the right thing?' I asked, scooping mashed raspberries from the depth of the glass with my finger. The disappointment of IUI had taken its toll. Plus, I was worried about money, conflicted about going private, conflicted about potential twins or triplets.

'Yes,' said Mark.

A drink or two later, in the toilets, swaying from the

alcoholic raspberries, I considered finger-swiping the cocaine traces from the mirrored sink-surround but reckoned I was hyped enough. At the bar, the pair of us drank and laughed, striving to enjoy ourselves, me jittery and verging on hysteria, and Mark, as usual, talking with his hands. Inevitably, he sent a drink flying.

We left before the bill reached three figures. It was just as well. Despite the detailed accounts, we had no idea what the process was going to cost us.

20

Somewhere between the waiting room and the ultrasound scan, I became reduced to my menstrual cycle and my reproductive organs. At home, I injected myself with hormones to quicken my ovaries until my thighs and belly were spotted with bruises. At the clinic, I became seriously intimate with the ultrasound probe, the little condom it wore and the slip of KY jelly. My egg follicles were slow to mature but I was swift to sense the disapproval of the doctors when my body didn't respond quite as quickly as expected.

Eventually, though, my eggs were ready for collection. When I came round from the anaesthetic, I was flabby-mouthed and excited, and told the anaesthetist that the anaesthetic was ace and that I was going to retrain in his specialty. In my delirium, I was convinced that he invited me to come to his house to learn.

Mark did his bit in private and his sample was prepped for the procedure. The embryologist called us to the lab. There was a problem. Under the microscope my eggs had a coating as thick as tractor tyres. For the sperm to penetrate, that coating would have to be punctured. That meant intracytoplasmic injection, the most unnatural version of this entirely unnatural process. It has increased risks. I couldn't let myself hear what the doctors were telling me.

A few days later clusters of cells were wobbling gently in a Petri dish. There were three embryos. The embryologist suggested they implant all three because my chances of pregnancy were low. My medical head said that for my own safety and the safety of the unborn children I shouldn't take the risk of triplets. My hormonal, desperate heart said I should take whatever chance I was offered. I agreed to all three.

The night of the implantation, I dream I am a goat, scrawny and manky, among a herd of cows who are round and maternal. I have little pink teats instead of comely udders. My pelvic bones jut through my wiry pelt. Like the doctor in the clinic, the farmer insists on fattening me up with milk from the cows. In real life, milk makes me retch and I struggle to keep it down. In my dream, it is unnatural and humiliating for a goat to be suckling from a cow. I am taken to a dark barn. The air in the barn is musty and scratches my throat. I feel an arm to its elbow inside me, and my cloven feet are scrabbling in the straw, but although my insides contract in pain, there are no baby goats to be tugged out of me, to membrane-slip between the farmer's fingers and land slimy and bloody in the straw for me to lick to life. Defeated, my goat-legs buckle underneath me. From outside the barn comes the contented lowing of the herd and their healthy calves as they are taken off to graze in meadows thick with sweet grass and clover. No such heavenly bliss for me. The farmer drags me by my four goat-ankles and loads me onto a bashed-up truck to be sold off cheap at the market.

★

The first time, it didn't work. They told me over the phone. I felt sick and stupid for trying. The second time, I have an appointment for the implantation the same day as an interview for a research fellowship in Glasgow. First thing in the morning, gazing down the microscope, I say hello to the two quivering embryos who might become my children before they are implanted, and then later the same morning, after the procedure, knickers back on, interview clothes readjusted, I dash along the road to the Wellcome Trust, where I will do my best to impress an expert panel with my research plan on the mechanisms of invasion of human red blood cells by the malaria parasite. A week or so later, I go off coffee and my ears ring with tinnitus. I don't dare hope. But when I phone for the result, they tell me it is positive.

Good girl, they say. As if I was a girl. As if I was good.

21

I let hope into my life and it all but destroyed me.

I was almost twelve weeks pregnant and approaching the first trimester scan, a safety line towards which I was anxiously crawling. We've got photos from that time, from a trip we took to Rye for a long weekend, where we stayed in a crooked Tudor hotel and bought a painting called *Two Sisters*, and I look different, even if the physical changes are not obvious. But in real life you could see a slight swelling round my tummy, and for once in my life I had boobs. Morning sickness was still a novelty. One Saturday trip to Borough Market and the smell of the cheese made me vomit. I felt special.

Much to my surprise, I had been awarded the Wellcome Trust fellowship and we were making plans to move to Glasgow. In August, we took a trip up there to search for houses. Among the ones we viewed was a beautiful, impractical ground-floor-and-basement conversion in a terrace off Great Western Road, with stained-glass panels above the door and a Wylie & Lochhead Arts and Crafts fireplace and matching bookshelves in the living room, which had once been the library. That room alone had more space than our entire London flat. A grand entrance hall, high ceilings, cast-iron radiators, windows that were taller than me, original floorboards – it was stunning. I let myself dream. I pictured us there. All three of us. Four, with the cat.

Once I'd established that the house had a tiny garden and a quiet lane out the back for the cat, I let myself worry about the impracticalities of heaving a buggy up and down the front steps, about the stairs coming off the kitchen, about the sharp corners on the fancy woodwork and whether it would be possible to make any of it baby-proof. We talked about nurseries and primary schools and didn't get far because it made us giggle. But we'd fallen for it, for the light and the heritage and the longing to be home.

Bids went to a closing date. Back in London, we debated and debated what we would be able to afford. Our finances had been ravaged after the IVF, but property prices in the capital had leapt since we'd bought our flat and we were about to double our money. We aimed high.

I was at work when Mark phoned the solicitor with our bid. He called me to let me know. She thought we had a good chance, he said, but it was impossible to say. My experiments that day were chugging along slowly. My back was aching. I was tired. I decided to duck home early and have a nap. I was half asleep when I got a text message from a friend. I told her I was at home.

'Why?'

'Back ache.'

'Anything else?'

'No. I'm fine.'

I didn't even think to read between the lines.

*

It is that same night. I can't sleep. I toss and turn for hours, thinking about the Glasgow house. At 3 a.m. I get up for a drink of water and go through to the living room to say hello to the cat. Sitting on the sofa in my vest and knickers, I cuddle her and whisper in her ear. We talk about Glasgow, about where we might live, about how I will still love her even when the baby comes. I go back to bed and drift in and out of anxiety.

When I wake in the morning, my knickers are soaking. In a panic, I swipe my hand between my legs but there is no blood. Maybe, I hope, maybe I just wet myself in my sleep. I get up and go to the loo. While I pee, I inspect my knickers. They are soaking. In the gusset, there is a glob or two of mucus. I pull toilet paper from the roll and wipe myself. The paper is stained with a tinge of pink.

'Mark,' I say. 'Mark.' I can't shout. I can't move. Black spots are crowding my vision.

'Did you call me?' Mark appears at the bathroom door. He sees I'm on the loo. 'Oh, sorry.' He almost turns to leave but catches my face. 'What? What is it? Helen, you're scaring me.'

'I think I'm losing the baby.'

He helps me up, leads me to the bedroom, calls the fertility clinic. They don't want to know. They have had their success. He calls our GP instead. We bag my wet knickers to show her. I dress slowly. Black t-shirt and khaki trousers. A little more than a year later, when I am soaked to the skin after walking hours in the rain, Mark will get those trousers out for me to change into but I will refuse to put them on. I will refuse to wear them ever again.

The GP says a bit of spotting is normal and not to

worry unless I start passing clots. We go home. Desperate to believe the GP, Mark does his best to reassure me, but I am certain the fluid in my knickers is amniotic fluid. It is only a matter of time.

When the clots start coming, we drive straight to the Whittington. It is the same hospital where I'd had round after round of unsuccessful IUI. As we cross the bridge over Highgate Hill, I feel a moment of stillness. Many metres below us, the world is carrying on as normal. Cars and delivery vans are scooting up and down the hill. Lorries and buses are fighting for space. Cyclists are jumping ahead at the traffic lights. The sounds of engines and the toots of horns. Shouts over the din of traffic. The roar of a motorbike. But here, time has stopped. It will all change when we walk through the hospital doors. I wonder if I should ask Mark to stop the car right there. If I should climb the iron railings to oblivion. Maybe it would be better to get it over with. I know what is coming. This pain is only the very start of it.

In A&E I am put on a trolley. A registrar reassures me that I am not necessarily having a miscarriage. But the contractions outdo even the worst of my endometriosis cramps and I am bleeding profusely. He is stalling for lack of beds.

Mark fusses around me. Lets me crush his hand when the pain is too much.

'What about your IVF drugs, your injections?'

'I don't know,' I say. 'I don't know if it is worth it any more.'

He asks a nurse. I am not officially having a miscarriage yet. He rushes off home to get the hormones. Helping in the only way he can think how.

While he is away, my blood pressure plummets. A sensation sweeps through me. It sweeps over and around me and blurs the staff rushing to and fro, but I can see the frightening figures on the monitor screen in close-up, acutely focused. I see myself sprawled on a trolley in a chaotic A&E, haemorrhaging dangerously but too weak to attract anyone's attention. Finally, the automatic blood-pressure monitor kicks in and someone hears its insistent alarm.

'Quickly. Cross match. Two units O neg.'

I finally get admitted.

I was right about the lack of beds. Mark finds me on an orthopaedic ward, zonked after pethidine shots. He comes armed with my injections and my toothbrush. I am due to have a scan the following morning and until then, there is still a level of hope. Or at least a level of pretence. The nurses are busy. I do my injections myself.

When he is chucked out, Mark takes my soiled clothes and leaves me sitting in bed in my hospital gown and paper knickers, clutching my knees and staring blankly at the opposite wall. At about 11 p.m., using my drip stand as a walking aid, I hobble to the bathroom to clean my teeth and go to the loo. I sit on the toilet, hunched over in pain and grief. By now the thick pad I am wearing is full not just of blood but of a pulpy mess of clots and dead tissue. In my drug haze, I pick some of it from the pad thinking maybe the doctors will want to do tests to find out what has gone wrong. It is sticky and formless. I pick another bit. Hold it between my fingers. Study it. And I see it. A tiny baby shape, not much bigger than a kidney bean. And my fingers are squeezing where its head should be. I panic. The bathroom whirls around me. The walls encroach. The tiles spin and blur. How could I have been so careless? I have squashed my baby's head. I have squashed my baby's head! What kind of monster am I? Distraught, I yank the pad from my knickers and place the baby bean into its centre. The toilet lid clatters behind me. I stagger out into the ward, searching for the night staff, dragging my drip stand with one hand, cradling the pad with the other. I don't know what I should do with it. How best to preserve it for tests. Eventually I find a nurse. She takes the pad from me and drops it in the clinical waste. Dumps my baby in the bin. So that is that. It is a first miscarriage. There will be no tests.

The next morning, I have a scan. In the darkened room, the white noise of the ultrasound resolves into boulders and caves. There is no flicker of a heartbeat to be seen. No sign of any pregnancy. Mark holds my hand and I think he cries, but I can't bear to witness his pain. I am numb. The nurse practitioner who had been in charge of my IUI spots me in the scan room. She knows without asking. She wraps me in her arms and her gorgeous, generous hug squeezes a few tears out of me.

We didn't get the Glasgow house. We missed out by a few thousand. The solicitor said she was sorry. Mark was gutted, mainly for me. But I was glad. I couldn't have lived in a house haunted by dreams.

22

The move to Glasgow came upon us before either of us was ready. I had sunk into grief. Mark did everything he could to protect me from having to deal with the logistics. We even bought a house without viewing it. I don't think I ever properly acknowledged what he was going through at the time. I don't think I was capable of letting myself. I was too damaged to add his pain to mine. But in the years that followed, whenever I saw him jiggling friends' kids on his knee, playing with our nieces and nephews, fooling around and getting them hyper before they went to bed (much to the delight of whoever was attempting to settle them for the night), sadness would stab deep in the centre of my heart and twist itself there.

The movers came to pack up the house while I was at the lab. At work, I emptied out my freezer space, packed up samples to send to Glasgow, boxed up lab books and files of results.

I told no one other than my boss what had happened. Disregard or not understanding the weight of my loss would have left me broken, but sympathy would have destroyed me entirely. My closest work friends had already left. Work was not the place it had once been. Perhaps because I was not the person I had once been. No one was allowed close enough to see the cracks in my plastered smile.

When I got home, all the furniture and most of our belongings had gone. All that remained could fit into a couple of large suitcases. My parents came to help with the last of it. That night we left the cat alone in the empty flat while we stayed in a grubby hotel nearby. I slept fitfully, dreaming of hospitals and babies. The next morning, while Mark stowed the last of our belongings in the car, I sat on the floor in the kitchen, leaning against the door to the boiler cupboard, with the cat wrapped tightly in my arms, fat teardrops rolling down my face, under my jawbone and dribbling down my neck. For once the cat stayed still in my arms and let me smother her with love.

'That's everything,' Mark called from the front door. I dragged myself to my feet and the cat leapt free. She headed towards the cat flap but I caught her. She yowled. I kissed the top of her head.

'Sorry, catkins,' I said as I shoved her, squirming, into her travel box. She would miss it here. The flat had been easy for her. Safe. Our tiny garden backed on to a lane with another set of gardens behind, so she had never wandered onto the busy roads.

Mark took the cat box to the car. Her howls of protest could be heard halfway along the street. I stood for a moment in the kitchen, staring at the wonky tiles we had tiled ourselves, remembering the excitement we'd felt when we had first moved in and the laughs we had had there with family and friends – dancing in the living room with my nieces wearing my luminous green netball knickers over their jeans, watching fireworks at Ally Pally from the back garden, nipping upstairs to party with our first-floor neighbours or to feed their fish when they were on their holidays, the cat as a kitten jumping into the middle of our Friday-night pizza at the start of her love affair with cheese. Christmases. Real summers. But we were going back home to Scotland. The shouts from the Territorial Army barracks, the overflowing, fox-mangled bin bags that spilled out of front gardens, the clip and glare of police helicopters, black snotters when we ventured into the depths of the city – in other circumstances, perhaps I wouldn't have asked myself if we were doing the right thing.

All at once I was overcome. The cry of the cat indistinguishable from the cry of an infant. The sensation that my baby was calling was overwhelming. Its spirit was there. It didn't want me to leave it behind. I had this urge to reach out and pick my baby up, to lift it by its underarms and feel the wriggle and the unexpected weight of it, to clasp it to my chest and never let it go. I wanted to kiss the smooth, cool skin of its cheek, squeeze its chubby limbs, bury my nose into its milky hair. My medical head told me that it was my hormones running wild – prolactin, oxytocin, both raised after the pregnancy – but I was frightened how deep inside me the desire ran. I reached out but my arms had withered.

Love lay down beside me and we wept.

Glasgow

23

It wasn't quite the triumphant return to Scotland that we had anticipated. We'd bought a beautiful house that was far too big for the two of us. A house I didn't belong in. A house I didn't deserve. The clouds were low, literally and metaphorically, and I was crushed under the weight of them.

Glasgow was home, but the city and I took a while to settle back to our old ways. It treated me the way of a jilted lover. It wasn't going to take me back with open arms when I had chosen to leave it. To many I was a stranger, my English side more evident than my Scottish side. The discovery that I had lived there before, that it was the blood of half of me, made it appear as if I had tried to hide the Scottish part of me when I had moved away. It wasn't true. My accent had always been fairly neutral, the Cumbrian vowels of my childhood sanded down for comprehension when we moved north. At work, the strain of hiding my grief came over as standoffishness. There was a clear assumption, or so I convinced myself, that with my Oxford degree I thought myself better than my colleagues. And I didn't have the wherewithal to act to refute this.

In the departmental lunchtime lectures, I sat in the

front row so as not to see the crowds behind me. Trained in the gladiatorial seminars of Oxford, I forced myself to ask questions, to be involved, to make my academic mark, to justify my fellowship and my position. But it portrayed a level of confidence that I didn't feel. At the occasional work event, I drank beer out of a bottle rather than a glass to hide the tremor that I couldn't control.

I was lucky, though. I might not have been capable of making new friends, but I still had many of my oldest, dearest friends around me.

'How's work going, H?' someone asked one Saturday night when a group of us were eating at our place.

I stabbed my fork into my chicken curry. 'OK, I guess. A bit tough. Setting up a new lab . . . You know.'

'What about the people you work with?'

'Yeah, they seem nice. Really nice. But I don't think they like me. It feels like a massive effort. I don't know if it's just me or not . . .' I tailed off. The others carried on eating. 'Serious question here, right. When you guys meet someone for the first time, is your natural assumption that they can't stand you?' They all looked up from their plates to see if I was being serious. 'I guess not,' I said. 'It's just me, then.'

And there were tears. Tears that wouldn't stop.

24

The receptionist led me to the consulting room. Effectively a made-over living room in what had been somebody's house, this was a space designed for baring one's soul in comfort. Lavender curtains protected the interior from intrusive daylight. In the corner, a lamp with a lavender shade cast a gentle glow on the matching walls. On the side table a bowl of potpourri was pretending to be dead rose petals but I could smell old-lady wardrobe sachets off it, so it didn't fool me. The receptionist encouraged me to relax while she fetched her colleague. I slumped into the sofa. The cushions plumped up around me, engulfing me in their lavender embrace. Soft music enveloped me. I swear it was lavender too.

I thought I had come to a local miscarriage charity for counselling. It appeared, however, that I had pitched up in relaxation hell. And I was about to be smothered alive.

The counsellor, when she arrived, was clutching a pad of paper to her chest. She smiled at me but I didn't smile back. It seems I had forgotten how. Instead, I looked her up and down and waited. I had fully expected her to be lavender too, but her cardigan diverged from the colour scheme. Nevertheless, the navy toned well with the painted walls and, together with the lamplight, gave her skin a bluish glow not far off the colour I had foreseen. She introduced herself as Margaret, scribbled something on the pad, which I imagine was my name, and asked me – when I was ready – to tell her a bit about what had happened.

'I had a miscarriage,' I said. It was obvious. Like the colour scheme.

She nodded gravely, unperturbed by my abrupt response. But she wanted more.

'After IVF.' Against my will, my words fissured with grief.

She smiled gently and took my hand. Offered words of condolence. Squeezed my fingers. She was in her element.

I was suffocating on empathy. I snatched my hand away.

Almost imperceptibly, she bristled. I was clearly very upset, she declared knowledgeably.

'And here's me thinking I was jumping for joy,' I said. My dart of sarcasm hit the wire. With sympathy oozing from her, she told me how she understood my hostility and my anger. Those emotions were common. They were a sign of grief and of feeling alone in my sadness. And of guilt.

'Guilt doesn't come into it.' I wasn't having anyone laying this at my door, tricking me into thinking it was all my fault.

Her compassion was making me nauseous.

'Do you know what?' I said. 'This is a mistake.'

She asked me to give the process a chance. Assured me that it would help. That talking and sharing were critical for recovery, and told me how many other women in my situation the charity had helped. Miscarriage was difficult – especially the first one – but it was common. And, she assured me, lots of women had miscarriages and went on to have families.

'You don't understand,' I said.

'Oh, but I do,' she said. Like all the counsellors here, she explained, she had had her own experience of miscarriage. She could relate exactly to what I was going through.

'It will get better,' she said. 'You're young. You have plenty of time to have the precious family that you want.'

'You aren't listening,' I said, shouting above the deafening roar of her gratuitous optimism. 'You are not listening.' Plus, she had made the sloppy mistake of assuming that my youthful countenance was a measure of actual youth. In the universal scheme thirty-five might pass as young, but in baby-making terms it was edging on Jurassic, even for a woman without my medical history.

'I *am* listening,' she insisted. 'I'm here to listen. You can say whatever you need to say. Don't be afraid to open up.'

'What's the fucking point?' I mumbled, more to myself than to her. I felt stupid. I had known it would be a waste of time. But it didn't lessen the disappointment that there was no way to fix this.

She implored me not to be so pessimistic, to have hope, to take comfort from the positive outcomes of all the other women who had been through the same as me.

'What?'

'Take comfort from the women who have been through the same—'

'Jesus fucking Christ,' I screeched. The lavender lampshade flinched. I wanted to snatch her clipboard and smash it over her stupid head. 'It isn't the same at all. I've had

IVF. I've got endometriosis. Infertility. I might not have another fucking chance.'

The poor woman looked at me aghast. There was a moment of silence. The curtains twitched. The lamp stuttered. The potpourri crumbled.

I picked up my belongings and fled.

25

An email arrived from Oxford with a dire warning in the subject line. 'Don't open this message unless you can go straight home.' The news it contained knocked me sideways. A close friend, one of the junior squash league, had died. A thrombotic stroke. The type you get from high blood pressure, obesity, smoking. It made no sense. She was the fittest person I knew.

I managed her funeral, but once it was over, I couldn't speak. Afterwards Mark and I went to Skye for a week. The first day it was sunny. We walked the Quiraing under a glorious blue sky. The rest of the week the cloud came down. The horizontal rain battered against the hotel window. I was glad. The dazzle of the sun burned my broken heart.

Back home, I had almost stopped functioning. My grief had mutated. Grown tentacles. Taken a grip of every part of me. I recognised it from before. The agitation, the insomnia, the thick lump of nausea wedged in my gullet. It had wheedled its way into my head. On repeat, its hideous refrain – I was useless, worthless, weak. A fraud. A joke. A waste of space. And I recognised that feeling too. That feeling that I wanted it all to stop.

My GP put me back on antidepressants. I smiled and said I was better. The psychiatric registrar saw through me and upped the dose. I think she recognised herself in me. She gave me her phone number and a book that had helped her. I read the book but didn't phone. She was about to cross a line in the way that I was prone to and I had to save her from herself. And from me.

I survived a year. The anniversary almost killed me.

26

A bloke in skinny black trousers and a baggy t-shirt ushered us in. His hair hung limply over his eyes. In a thin voice, he introduced himself as Scott. He left us in a side room with beige vinyl chairs, where we sat studying the cracked grey linoleum. A few moments later, he re-appeared with weak tea in polystyrene cups.

'Toast?' he asked.

'Er, no thanks,' Mark said.

'Your room will be ready soon,' he promised.

Mark held my hand as we waited in silence.

'I'm not staying here,' I said eventually.

'Helen, we've been through this . . .'

'I'm not staying.'

'You have a choice,' the social worker told me when she arrived on the ward. 'You can stay here of your own free will, or we will section you.'

'That's not a fucking choice,' I said.

I waited until she had gone before I told the nurse in charge that I was leaving.

'You can't,' she said.

'You can't fucking stop me,' I said.

'Yes, I can.' As she was happy to elucidate, under Section 25 (2) of the Mental Health Act (Scotland), she had the right to detain me for up to two hours until a doctor could see me to take it further. Which she did. It was my first taste of what it meant to have my freedom taken from me. It was a sour taste of disbelief and rage, and it was a taste I would come to know well.

When the room was ready, Mark was sent home. Scott took me through to see it, hovering at the door while I looked around. There was a bed with a thin, worn quilt, a bedside cabinet made of cheap wood laminate and a small sink with a mirror above it. Behind a sliding door in the corner was a toilet. It had not been cleaned.

I looked in the mirror and tried smiling. Red-rimmed eyes with black circles stared back at me.

I sat on the edge of the bed and the walls closed around me.

Two days later I finally crawled out of my room and went to watch the TV in the sitting room. The room was almost full with patients who all seemed to know one another. I sat down on an empty chair. There was a collective gasp.

'Aargh, you bitch, get off my pal,' a lad said, his eyes flashing as he lunged for me. Scott leapt from his armchair and pulled him off me. I found out later he was called Davy.

'Nutter,' I mumbled. The others sniggered and went back to watching *Bargain Hunt*. I hauled myself up and dragged myself back to my room. I could hear Davy arguing over the empty seat.

Scott followed me and parked himself on the chair outside my room. I slammed the door shut and sat on the bed. He pushed the door open.

'You know the rules,' he said gently.

But that was the thing. I had no idea about the rules.

At the ward round the following day, Dr Lorimer asked me how I was.

'Fine,' I said. He laughed.

'That's the thing about Helen,' he said to Priti, his registrar. 'She's always fine.'

Priti suited her name with her sleek black hair and delicate features. In keeping with the latest fashion, she wore her stethoscope slung casually around her neck. Her brown woollen trousers were slightly too big for her, and the sleeves of her fine-knit sweater were always tugged down over her hands. Her ingenuous appearance belied her forensic eye. I would never succeed in getting one past her.

'When can I go home?' I asked.

'I don't think we are even considering that yet,' Dr Lorimer replied. His hair fluffed up in panic.

'Oh, for fuck's sake,' I said. 'I am perfectly fucking fine.' I wasn't the one wearing an ill-fitting tweed jacket with elbow patches and diarrhoea-coloured jumbo cords.

'I don't think so, Helen,' he said.

I wasn't fine, that much was clear, but I didn't understand what was happening to me. None of it was new: the grief, the depression, the constant criticism inside my head. But I had stopped being able to deal with it. After a year of putting up a front, a lifetime of trying to be someone better, after my hope to be someone different had died with my baby, I had felt something give inside. The drive that had kept me going had snapped.

I couldn't do it any more. I was tired. Tired of the expectations I put on myself. Tired of whatever it was that had decreed that I had to be perfect. Tired of the judgement – my own internal judgement and the judgement I had externalised – whenever I fell short. Tired of having to try so hard all the time.

I was tired of everything.

Tired of myself.

Tired of life.

I met Craig, my first named nurse, at the ward round. He was supposed to be the one with overall care of me. He was a fair bit younger than me, but it didn't stop him addressing me like an errant adolescent. Mind you, with his precise side parting and his dinner-plate glasses, he seemed to be doing his utmost to pass as middle-aged. He even sported a navy blazer over his uniform-regulation, pale-blue polo shirt.

After the ward round was finished, he barged into my room with a smirk across his face.

'Your solicitor is coming tomorrow,' he said in a weedy, nasal voice.

'What solicitor?'

'For your court case next week.'

'What court case?'

He didn't bother to explain.

We were supposed to have one-to-one sessions where I told him what I was feeling. It was meant to help, to give me some kind of release.

'Craig, I think you are a prick,' I told him.

'I don't give a fuck what you think,' he told me in reply.

That may have been the case but it didn't stop him

making a monumental effort to live down to my opinion of him.

For three days, the nurses brought my drugs to my room. After that, I was made to queue like everyone else. The drug trolley barred the entrance to the treatment room to protect the nurse on duty from the mob. The first time it was Isobel, the ward manager, with Les as her bouncer to keep us in line. He was a nursing assistant who moonlighted as a stand-up comedian. But I could never find the comedy in him. Not in his muscles chiselled from granite nor even in the straggly grey ponytail that tickled his collar.

Isobel dished the drugs out in miniature plastic beakers. I took mine to go back to my room.

'Where do you think you're going?' Les yelled. I froze. Someone in the queue signalled to me. Isobel beckoned me back to the trolley and poured me a cup of water. 'You take them here.'

The surface of the water rippled in my trembling hand. I took each tablet. Gulped. Swallowed.

'Mouth.'

She checked under my tongue and in the pouches of my cheeks. Nodded to let me go.

I slunk back to my room without looking at the queue. I had learned already that such happenings were what passed as entertainment in that place.

There was nowhere to hide. Twenty-four hours a day the staff were in my face. Constant observation meant the toilet door had to be left open, the shower door left unlocked, with check calls I had to echo back, footsteps a pace or two behind me wherever I went. Even if I had made a run for it, I wouldn't have been able to escape. The front door was locked to me. In bed, day or night, I would roll onto my side, presenting an expressionless back to my captors so they wouldn't perceive my night terrors, my weakness, my tears.

Within a week I lost what remained of my appetite. Meal times were a torment. All I ate was soup the colour of insipid pond water with bloated lumps of barley floating in it. The other food was worse. Grey, boiled potatoes served with chunks of gristle in slimy gravy. Vegetables so overcooked they had lost all identifying features. Sickly sponge pudding and custard that smelled of bad eggs. I lost weight and considered myself supermodel thin.

At the queue for dinner one evening Scott asked me how I was doing.

'Don't ask them that, sonny,' said Laugh-a-Minute Les. 'If you ask them that, they'll think you give a shit.'

The psychologist I had seen a few times in the past came to visit me in hospital. Out in the real world, we'd rubbed along fine. But when he arrived on the ward, he took me into a consulting room at the far end, away from the nursing staff and other patients, and there, in the semi-darkness, with the curtains half-drawn, surrounded by the bulky armchairs making a clumsy attempt at comfort, he questioned me. He wanted to ascertain exactly how I had ended up being admitted. From where I was sitting, though, it felt like an interrogation. As if being in hospital was my personal failing for which he was being held responsible.

Pinned to the shit-brown sofa by nausea and etiquette, I squeezed myself further and further into the corner, folding in on myself, trying to disappear. After half an hour, there was nowhere else to retreat. I felt like a cornered animal, injured and whimpering. All I wanted was for it to stop so I could go back to my room and hide. Against my better judgement, I agreed to have more sessions with him.

'Good,' he said, lifting his briefcase from the coffee-ringed table. He stood up, drew himself to his full height. 'I'll make arrangements with the team.'

I glanced at him. I could feel panic snarling under my skin.

'Actually, no,' I said. 'I've changed my mind. Please, please just leave me alone.'

'Now you're being silly.'

It was too much. I lost it. I screamed at him. Swore. Told him to leave me the fuck alone. I didn't want his therapy or any of his other type of torture.

'You are being ridiculous,' he said, backing away from me. 'You clearly need help.'

'Fuck off. Fuck off. Fuck the fuck off.' I was screeching, wailing, blocking my ears with my fists. My screeches must have travelled the length of the corridor because Lorraine, the charge nurse, came running to the rescue.

'OK, enough,' she said. 'You.' She beckoned him and, to the amusement of the day room, escorted him to the front door where, ignoring his protests that I'd agreed to treatment, informed him in no uncertain terms that he would not be coming back. I trailed behind her, more bedraggled than ever. At the time I thought it was me who Lorraine had rescued but, looking back, I realise that perhaps it was him.

★

The court hearing was the following week.

The courthouse had a magnificent marble foyer that echoed with the footsteps of solicitors, but the courtroom was nothing more than a seminar room with several rows of plastic chairs and no windows. The sheriff listened to Dr Lorimer's testimony.

'Do you have anything to add, Dr Taylor?' he asked. I shrugged my shoulders. The proceedings were a joke as far as I was concerned and, but for the chance of a day out, I would have refused all part in the rigmarole. The sheriff made his ruling under Part V, Section 18 of the Mental Health Act (Scotland) and I was formally detained for six months, subject to renewal, as laid out in Section 30 of the aforesaid Act.

I left the courtroom with a nurse on either side of me. As we stood outside in the drizzle waiting for a taxi, I watched the treacly water of the Clyde flowing past and wondered how cold it would be.

27

'Kinda daft, isn't it?' I said. We were in a taxi on our way to the Western Infirmary. Elspeth winked at me and made one of her eyebrows dance. We both sniggered. Hers was the throaty gurgle of a smoker. I liked her, and not just because she laughed at my sick jokes. In other circumstances, we might have been friends. She was about my age, maybe a bit younger. The twists on her uniform, like her black Adidas trainers and her thick eyeliner, showed her for the indie kid she had once been. Her hair was dark brown, almost black, and straight to the point of snapping, and she wore her long fringe plastered to the side and had to peer out from under it. She treated me like a human being and was one of the few who had been willing to accompany me out of the ward for my appointment. One of the few prepared to take the risk.

This was my first legitimate visit outdoors, bar the trip to court, and it was to have a breast lump biopsied. The lump I'd first noticed in the car back from the airport on the way home from holiday several months earlier. The seat belt had rubbed uncomfortably on the upper edge of my right breast and I thought perhaps I'd pulled a muscle. Closer examination revealed a definite lump. I wasn't particularly alarmed. I'd had one removed two years earlier in the midst of all the tests and minor surgeries around the investigation for my infertility. That one had been a benign lump of no consequence. Nevertheless, Mark insisted I get this one checked out. The GP sent me to a clinic. The clinic organised a biopsy. The appointment for the biopsy arrived after I had been admitted.

At the breast clinic, I sat on an examination trolley naked from the waist up, with my legs hanging over the side, dripping with anxiety despite the relative cool of the clinic. The hiss of blood-pressure monitors, the clank of weighing scales, the squeal of trolley wheels echoed off the sterile walls. Instruments clattered into steel bowls and through my bones. Voices were too strident, the buzz of fluorescent lights too loud, the bulbs too bright. There was a hideous possibility of meeting someone I knew from medical school, someone now promoted and successful, someone who would look at me and struggle to recognise me. To keep the panic from overtaking me, I hung my head and focused on my half-naked body. My stomach had caved in, my hip bones jutted over the top of my jeans, my ribs stood out like a desert skeleton.

'Can you sit up straight, please?'

I hadn't heard the specialist arrive. She was someone I knew vaguely. A friend of a sister of one of my friends. That was already a relationship too close. I grabbed the underside of the trolley beside my knees to keep my tremor under control and sat up as straight as I could while she assessed me from a short distance, looking for unevenness or skin puckering or changes to my nipples. She examined my armpits, checking for lymph nodes.

'Sorry.'

'What for?'

'Sweat.' I was dissolving in shame at my uncooperative body.

She didn't reply.

'It's worth being cautious,' she said a little later, as she stuck the biopsy needle into the lump, 'but I'm pretty sure this isn't anything to be alarmed about.' She had mistaken my shakiness and anguish for dread about the outcome. She peered at me, expecting signs of relief, and seemed a touch put out when they didn't come.

It was raining when we left the clinic. Byres Road was dark. Car tyres swished along the wet road, headlights blurred to coronas by the rain. Elspeth swore when she saw the weather.

'We'll have to run,' she said. 'I don't have a brolly.'

'We won't get that wet.' I was trying to sound casual. 'It's not like it's tanking down.' We had come out of an exit directly behind the university laboratories where I should have been doing my research. The idea of encountering a work colleague was making me almost physically sick but fear and vertigo had me rooted to the spot. The growl of traffic, the reek of diesel and wet tarmac, the whiff of takeaways piled on the nausea. Home-time workers and hunched pedestrians stepped around me, but I felt crowded and unsteady. Any second, I was going to collapse, merge in a blob with a puddle. I needed to take it slowly, adjust to the evening rush, navigate the crowds. I was counting on the darkness and the weather to shroud me. Plus, the taxi rank was up beside the Underground station and I wasn't convinced my legs would run the distance.

'Come on. Let's go.' Elspeth was getting impatient.

'Do we have to?'

'Yes, we have to,' she said. 'Or we will have a catastrophe on our hands.'

I had no idea what she was going on about, but she had already set off. I stepped out into the seething night. Ahead, she paused under a street light.

'Move it, missus,' she shouted against the weather.

'On you go,' I shouted back. 'I'll make my own way home.'

She laughed and ran ahead to hail a taxi.

Inside the black cab, bolstered by the relative warmth and the stiff upholstery, I wiped the drizzle off my glasses and asked her what she'd meant.

'My hair,' she said.

Turned out that her hair wasn't straight after all. It was delinquently curly and she detested it. Every morning she straightened it to three times its natural length and plastered it flat with enough hair lacquer to be a fire risk when she smoked. Which meant she had to be vigilant. And avoid the damp at all costs.

It was crazy. To live in Glasgow and hope that you could avoid the damp seemed as futile and deluded as the most extreme of my self-deceptions.

The biopsy results came back a few days later. As expected, the lump was benign. I felt no relief. If anything, a tinge of disappointment. I didn't particularly want to die of cancer, but at least it would have taken the effort out of killing myself.

28

Weeks passed. There were no more trips outside. I spent hours staring out the window of my room – a window that was reinforced glass and that wouldn't open more than a couple of centimetres – plugged in to my CD player or my radio, listening to the music of British Sea Power and Johnny Cash, or John Peel's soothing voice. I watched scurrying commuters take a shortcut past the wards to the train station at the end of the road, and the dog walkers wandering freely on the grassy slopes of the old hospital grounds. The old Victorian asylum was shut down now, the windows boarded up and the walls vandalised. I'd been taught there as a medical student. There was talk that it was to be converted to luxury flats. I wondered who would buy one.

I wrote. Pages and pages of unreadable torment in a hard-backed journal that a friend had given me a year earlier to chart my pregnancy and the birth of the child that didn't come. And I read. Eliot, Thackeray, Tolstoy. Different worlds, different times.

My meetings with Dr Lorimer bristled with mutual exasperation.

'It isn't healthy, keeping me locked up,' I said. 'I need fresh air.'

'We can't risk it at this stage, I'm afraid.'

He tried every kind of antidepressant and more on me.

'You do know, don't you,' I said, 'that just because I want to kill myself, it doesn't make me a fucking nutter.'

'That kind of language isn't helpful, Helen.'

The stale air of the ward settled in my lungs and mouldered my brain. I kept to my single room whenever I could. In the morning, I took my shower in the bathroom along the corridor from my room before anyone else was up. Breakfast was a hurried affair, where I shielded myself with muteness. Lunch, if I bothered, was solitary. To avoid the queue, I went as late as I could and ate alone. When visitors came, they sat with me in my room rather than the communal spaces. Those days, for the drug round, I waited until the last possible minute, preferring to be rounded up by Laugh-a-Minute Les with his casual insults than face the queue, face having other patients encroach upon my space and, in the spirit of harmless enquiry, check out what meds I was on. I didn't want to have to explain myself.

Wherever I went, I looked downwards and inwards. I didn't want to look up, I didn't want to look around me. I was afraid of what I would see. I was afraid I might catch my reflection in a window or mirror or in the demeanour of other patients. Afraid of accepting what was happening to me, afraid of accepting that I was there to stay and afraid what the other patients would think if they knew how cushy my life was.

*

Billy, a patient with alcoholic dementia and a vicious line in obscenities, liked to torment me for sport. Or so I was convinced. Whenever he was in, he'd beat me to the shower in the morning and pee all over the floor and the tiles, and play the confusion card if I dared to pass comment. If I wanted to shower, I was left with no choice. With my guards outside, you would find me down on my hands and knees, wiping up Billy's piss with blue paper towels and skooshing the floor with water, trying and failing to get rid of the reek without cleaning product. I was so lost, so fearful, that I never thought to ask anyone for help.

29

Weeks slipped into months. The vigil at my window was unabating. I was unable to tear myself away. I'd wait for Dr Lorimer to appear around the corner of the old hospital and take the path down the slope to Ferguson House, trying to divine from the spring in his step or the drag of his heels whether or not his visit to the ward was to see me. I wanted the constant observation to be lifted. I wanted to go outside. Although I was frantic to see him, his presence on the ward agitated me. If he saw me and nothing had changed, my fury erupted and left me spent, but if he left without seeing me, I was wrung out with despair. I hated how needy and annoying I had become. At long last, though, fresh air was sanctioned. The permission, when it came, was unexpected. It swept away my resentment and drowned me with gratitude. My rage had been compromised.

Stepping outside for the first time in months was as exotic and unfamiliar as stepping off the plane in The Gambia had been when I went there to work as a medical student. Except this time, instead of a head-on collision with a wall of heat, here were grey clouds kneading my head and lichen-tinged dampness clinging to my skin. I sat on the bench beside the front door, sandwiched between Staff Nurse Naveed and Newly Qualified Nicola, blinking against the grey daylight and drinking in the wet-leaf smell. In the ward my senses had become lazy. The clang of hammer and anvil in my eardrums had been dampened by the sameness of the hospital sounds. Outside, the clatter of trains made me flinch and the raucous chat of magpies made me twitch. With my heightened senses, each whisper of breeze bit my face and made me wince. And each flinch, each twitch, each wince, engendered an equal and opposite reaction in my sentries. Ready to chase me should I flee.

Patients with outdoor privileges hung around the entrance smoking and chatting, waiting for lifts to their temporary freedom or for their drinking pals to accompany them to their AA meetings. The atmosphere was convivial, relaxed. They regarded me with curiosity. Most of them hadn't encountered me at such close proximity before. The months of being an inpatient had rubbed the edge off my ignorance, but the outdoor patients were still much more sussed than I was. Out here, flanked by Naveed and Nicola, my situation was evident. These patients knew the system well enough to know exactly what this meant. I was a flight risk and a suicide risk.

'Hey, doll,' someone said. 'Got a light?'

Months of confinement had laid waste to my conversational skills. Before my agitation engulfed me in flames, Naveed stepped in with his lighter to save me.

We had barely settled on the bench when Isobel, the ward manager, stuck her head out of the door. 'Naveed, can you do the meds, please? Helen, that's all for today.'

'You're kidding me.' The cold of the damp wooden

bench hadn't even had the time to seep through my jeans. I looked wildly at Naveed. 'A bit longer. Please.'

But Naveed was needed elsewhere and, as a recent graduate, the deal with Newly Qualified Nicola was they wouldn't leave me alone with her until I had demonstrated that I could be trusted. Almost weeping, I was escorted back inside.

30

Christmas arrived and I was still under constant observation and often stuck inside the ward. Dr Lorimer decided he would allow me out for four hours on Christmas Day. Mark came to collect me. I changed out of my ripped jeans and faded sweatshirt into a red dress that hung like a sack on me. At home, I watched the clock and cried into my M&S turkey breast with cranberry sauce. When the time was up, Mark took me back to the ward.

On Boxing Day, I absconded.

For once, the staff outnumbered the patients. Ferguson House was empty bar those poor souls with nowhere to go and the couple of us that they wouldn't let out. On Christmas evening, there had been a party in the television room, but I hadn't gone. I had nothing to celebrate. Lying on my bed staring at the ceiling, I had imagined Barbara, the activity nurse, in the TV room that she had decorated with tinsel and fake presents, hoping to persuade the others to pull crackers or join her as she sang carols while they watched bemused from the armchairs, too polite or too drugged to protest, drinking supermarket cola or imitation Irn Bru and waiting for her to get on with it so they could turn the television back on.

I had been traumatised by the visit home. The familiarity and the strangeness of the house where I was meant to live had unsettled me completely. It was disconcerting to go to the bathroom unobserved, to use handwash scented with pink grapefruit rather than disinfectant, to dry my hands on a towel that wasn't sandpaper rough and imbued with the smell of the hospital laundry. It was unsettling to be alone with my husband, to cuddle the cat and bury my face in her fur and feel the pinpricks of love wakening my emotions. The pressure of the ward had meant shutting down, numbness as a means to endure. Home lifted by inches that load, forced feeling to flow through my veins. I couldn't deal with its intensity, nor the excruciating rebound pain.

Back on the ward, I tried to oust thoughts of home from my mind by cramming it with junk. I played game after game of *Minesweeper* on an ancient computer in an unoccupied side room which was occasionally used for private meetings or therapy sessions. It was a graveyard of obsolete equipment, broken furniture and missing files. There were faulty printers, chairs with screws loose, outdated educational pamphlets unread and bleached by age. Later, I'd have the odd therapy session there. It meant perching on a wobbly chair or hauling in an armchair from the corridor. Sessions were overheard and discussed by the occupants of the smoking room next door. All your secrets and fears were fair game.

Late Boxing Day evening, when there was no space left for thought, I went back to my room, where Laugh-a-Minute Les was slouching on an armchair outside. I was considering going to bed when I heard the doorbell.

'Food,' Les said gleefully, and went off to collect the

delivery. I plonked myself on my bed and yanked off my trainers. Les returned laden with bags of carryout curry, which he immediately secreted in the staff room. One by one the night staff joined him. The window of the staff room gave on to the open workspace directly outside my room, and I watched their silhouettes – turned orange by the synthetic curtains – stooping over dishes and spooning curry onto plates. Shadow marionettes.

Puppeteers turned puppets. Opportunity clashed with confusion. There was no one on guard. Without my puppet masters, I was unstrung by nerves. I closed my door quietly and leaned against it to collect myself. For three months I'd been under constant observation, day and night. Without my guards I felt oddly exposed.

I was in a trance of indecision when voices outside made me start. I inched open the door. Billy and a man I didn't recognise passed by. They had unlit cigarettes pinched between their fingers. Strange, given they were coming from the direction of the smoking room. The whiff of opportunity suddenly got stronger. I crept out of my room and padded after them, hanging back in doorways and shadows, not daring to be seen, even by other patients. When they rounded the corner before the reception office, I hung back. From my hiding place, I distinctly heard the clatter of the front door flung wide and the guilty clunk of its rebound.

Could that be right? Had Billy and his mate really gone outside for a cigarette? I peered around the corner of the office. Through the wire-hatched window of the door, I could make out their smoking forms. I couldn't believe it. The ward was unlocked! Les had messed up. He hadn't locked it again after the delivery. Every muscle in my body began to quiver, every nerve started fizzing. The temptation to bolt was almost irresistible. Was anyone around to stop me? I veered into the TV room. Did a sweep for unremarked spies. No one. I sat down for a minute, head spinning, forgetting in my confusion to first check the sofa for the outpourings of Billy's incontinent bladder.

I wasn't wearing shoes. If I was going to do this, I needed more than socks on my feet.

Nonchalantly – pulse rattling, breath clattering – I made my way back to my room. The staff room door was still shut.

I put on my boots. Fastened the laces with thick, clumsy fingers. Took my Gore-Tex rain jacket from the locker. It was waterproof but thin, meant for summer showers and autumn drizzle, little use against the winter cold. But it could fold in on itself, fit into its own pocket, easy enough to hide if I shoved it up my jumper.

Outside, it was cold and drizzling. I crossed the road and hurried away from the ward, hugging the shelter of the overhanging trees and shaking the rain jacket free of its zipped pocket. I tugged it on. Enrobed in the black of it, I was swallowed by the dark. I walked quickly, but my actions belied the blankness of my thoughts. I didn't have a plan. Beyond getting away.

Once I was out of the hospital grounds, I headed up the main road. Sights I knew loomed like apparitions in the night rain: the school sports ground blurred by protective floodlights; the looming flats at Anniesland Cross, their balconies laden with blinking Santa sledges; the supermarket forecourt dead after the Christmas rush. Everything hazy and indistinct and rendered silent by the low cloud and the stress muffling my thoughts. I cut through the supermarket car park, down to the towpath beside the canal, and let it drag me where it wanted.

A while later I was shaken from my stupor by the toot of a train. Without realising, I had come as far as the station one stop from home. Between me and the train was a black ribbon of water that I'd hardly been aware of. Alert now, I scrambled over the footbridge spanning the canal. The train was pulling in to the station, its headlights ploughing two furrows through the drizzle. The platform was deserted, save a single passenger waiting to board. In the darkness, I watched the train draw to a standstill, the guard spring down from a rear carriage, a young lad hop off near the front. The weather was getting thicker, smothering the light from the open doors, extinguishing it before it could escape from the carriage. The boy took the cast-iron steps of the railway bridge two at a time and disappeared into the night. The guard waited, shrouded by the rainfall. For a moment, we shared the deserted platform. She turned away and climbed into a carriage up front. As the beeps signalled the closing doors, I jumped into the carriage she had just left.

I had no ticket and no money. If the guard came looking for me, I was done for. Twitchy and hypervigilant, I stood at the door, ready to dodge her rather than risk being cornered in a seat. Other passengers in the belly of the carriage were staring at me. It didn't take much to imagine what they were seeing: wild eyes, straggly hair, clothes hanging off me, pale and shaky. I stopped myself from staring them down.

Minutes later, we were passing my house. From the carriage, I could see the lights in the living-room window.

Mark was probably watching TV. The shelter of the house, the warmth of the light, the promise of safety were luring me home. But if I did go home, Mark would be forced to take me back to the ward and, thereafter, we would resent each other for what I had made him do.

The train pulled in to the station. Someone pushed past me to exit. Through the open doors I heard the guard calling goodnight to the driver. The rain was pelting hard. The guard hurried along the platform without giving me a second glance. The echoes of her footsteps were clipped short by the foul weather. Her shift was over. The doors beeped to close. I stepped back and took a seat. The train chugged on. Inertia and indecision had forced me onwards.

At the end of the line, I sneaked off the train and dodged past the ticket booth and the exit. But there was no one collecting tickets. From the car park, I took the underpass, which dipped below the main road and resurfaced near a bridge over a rain-swollen stream. I paused for a moment on the bridge, watching the water spill and gurgle beneath me. A fleeting thought bubbled below my consciousness, one that I hadn't been aware of when I'd been trudging along the steady canal. But the stream was too shallow to jump into and I was too cold to contend with the icy water. I wanted to die but, at that moment, I had neither the energy nor the inclination to take the plunge.

I set off into the freezing rain, unsure where I was headed. I pulled the flimsy hood out of the collar of my jacket and walked with purpose to convince myself that I had a plan. Alert and jumpy now, it was as if there was a short circuit in my brain. My thoughts were no longer dulled but they would not string themselves together. They looped past reason, the most superficial of them driving me on. The path trailed the edge of the river, along muddy tracks that backed on to vast gardens, tracked beside a children's play park, and I trailed with it until I reached the edge of open parkland and the start of the West Highland Way. It seemed as good a route as any.

At the entrance to the parkland, a group of youths were blocking my path. 'Merry Christmas,' I mumbled. They glanced at me and scuttered out of my way. I put my head down and carried on into the darkness. Rain was lashing down, sticking the hood to my head, plastering my hair to my face. It was pouring off the Gore-Tex below my waist, soaking my jeans around my bum and thighs. Water had begun to seep through my boots. The clatter of my chattering teeth could be heard above the storm.

Soon, the park opened on to moorland scattered with copses, which offered intermittent respite from the rain. Somewhere nearby there were Second World War bunkers and gun placements which would provide shelter until the rain let up. But I didn't come across them. The darkness and the weather had twisted paths I'd thought were straight.

After an hour I was frozen, exhausted and lost. For the previous three months I'd done nothing but sit in my room or lie in my bed. Today I had walked miles. A horizontal wind was driving the rain between the seams of my jacket. My fingers were stark white in the darkness, bloodless from clutching the flaps of my hood to keep the water from trickling down my neck. There was nothing left for my body to keep itself warm. I had completely given in to the cold. My teeth had stopped chattering. I was no longer shivering. Steel rods of cold had set deep in my bones.

I traipsed on, close to collapse, wandering out of the open heath of the country park and on to a back road. The road skirted cultivated woodland where the pine trees stood in regiments, unperturbed by the driving rain, densely packed enough for their spreading branches to cast a protective canopy over the forest floor. The trees were offering me shelter and peace. All I wanted to do was surrender to them, to curl up under their branches on that bed of dry needles, and sleep. And if I died of hypothermia during the night, so much the better.

There was a banking up to the low limestone wall that marked the boundary of the forest. It wasn't high, maybe three or four feet, but the slope was steep and slippery. Pre-Ferguson House, I would have managed it in a stride or two. But Ferguson House had depleted me. I scrambled halfway. Slipped down. Picked myself up. Tried again. Slipped. I could hardly see because of driving rain and tears. And again I tried, and again, until my hands were scraped and bleeding, and my clothes as muddy and slippery as the banking.

The slope was insurmountable. I collapsed onto my knees in the road and let the rivulets of rain run alongside me. I dammed the water with my hand until it ran over my fingers. I was too weak and pitiful even to cry.

The rain lashed down. The wind howled. The short circuits in my brain were no longer firing. The circulation had all but stopped in my fingers. My feet felt like they had been steamrollered. My face an ice-block, glacial against my whipping hair.

Eventually, I dragged myself up and trudged on, past farm fields and scattered houses. At length I came across a village I half knew. Without realising, I had looped around on myself. An unthinking defeat. My guts twisted. I thought I would vomit. The city stretched out below me in the distance, its sky a sickly globe of mustard gas. Police helicopters were scanning the vicious night, their searchlights slicing through the toxic glow of light pollution. I wondered who they were chasing.

By 2.30 a.m. I was outside my front door. The lights were still on in the living room but now their glow was ominous. I rang the doorbell. Mark opened the door. Behind him, one of our closest friends peered over his shoulder. They swept me in, helped me out of my wet clothes, ran me a hot bath. The heat stung my skin, fought and failed to penetrate below the surface, and left me red and scalded. Mark laid out dry clothes for me – the khaki miscarriage trousers, which I refused to wear – but then he found others and I pulled them on, resigned to my fate. When I was dressed, they hugged me tightly and let my tears soak into their shoulders. And then the police arrived.

Twenty minutes later I was back on the ward.

The following day Lorraine, my latest named nurse, asked me how I was doing. I fought back the tears that always spiked my eyes those days whenever someone was kind to me.

'Don't beat yourself up,' she said. 'You're going through a lot. Being on the ward isn't easy. Even for the folk who are used to it, it isn't exactly a walk in the park.'

'Last night it was,' I said. 'That's exactly what it was. A walk in the park.' We laughed but I wasn't sure it was funny.

'I hope you're not thinking of fucking off again,' Les said that evening. He was pissed off because he was in trouble for not keeping me under observation. 'What the hell were you playing at?'

I didn't reply. I didn't have an answer. Because I knew what he was thinking. I knew what everyone was thinking. All my talk of suicide was bullshit, wasn't it? If I really meant it, I'd be dead by now.

31

After my Boxing Day stunt, outdoor privileges were completely withdrawn. Once again, I was confined, reduced to staring numbly out of the window, my pain barely relieved by the kindnesses of Amanda and Gentle John, nursing assistants who ensured we always had clean sheets, who dug out the decent biscuits for the afternoon cuppy, who made toast if we hadn't managed the canteen slop.

Together with Barbara, the activity nurse, Gentle John was an avid disciple of the Atkins diet. On the days when John was guarding my door, Barbara would stop by to compare their daily egg and bacon input.

'You can eat as much as you like, you know,' she told me as if I was interested. 'So long as it is protein.'

During the week, Barbara ran relaxation classes that none of the patients attended. She'd skip round the ward in her yoga outfit trying to persuade us to participate, to bring our pillows and go into the sitting room, where the lights were dimmed and the TV turned off for once, to listen to whale song and Pan pipes. I always refused. It wasn't the escape I was looking for.

★

To pass the time, I started doing jigsaws. The more complicated the better. The close concentration required to search thousands of identically sized pieces of iceberg distinguished only by nuanced shades of white or to complete a cloudless, featureless sky left little room to listen to the endless accusations in my head that claimed there was nothing actually wrong with me. I kept searching for proof that I was ill, that I hadn't conned Dr L, that Laugh-a-Minute Les and all the other folk who I was sure had me down as a malingerer were wrong in their ignorant assessment. I needed reassurance that I was legit and not just slacking. According to Mark, Dr L had said I was the worst case of depression he had ever seen, but I reckoned that at least one of them was havering. Looking back, though, if there is one objective measure that proves beyond a shadow of a doubt that I really was ill – that I was *really* ill – it was this fondness for jigsaws.

For light relief, Lorraine told me stories of the more unusual ways patients had tried to kill themselves. A man had tried to poison himself by eating rhododendrons. He'd sustained twig-related injuries but nothing life-threatening. One woman, she said, had tried to cut her wrists with a Quaver. We came to the conclusion, as did the woman, that corn snacks were not the most effective way of ending one's life.

Lorraine was Dr Lorimer's eyes and ears on the ward. At forty, she was only four years older than me, but she had married as a teenager and was the mother of four grown-up sons – a background that I'm sure influenced her approach to work. She was fierce, funny and protective, and I always imagined her as a mother lion and us, staff and patients alike, as her cubs to be taken care of (and kept under control should the need arise). It was an impression that was reinforced if you ever saw her patrolling the ward, striding up and down the corridors with her thick plait swishing wildly behind her.

Being under constant obs was almost tolerable if it was Lorraine on duty. Though she spent most of that time sitting outside my room reading gossip magazines, almost nothing escaped her. She spotted the wounds in my marriage and tried to bandage them.

'Mark had no choice but to bring you back,' she said. 'You know that, right?' I didn't have the words to answer. 'And he had no alternative but to agree to your section.'

When she had read all she could about Gwyneth Paltrow's wedding or Britney Spears' bikini body, she'd come into my room and regale me with outrageous stories, sometimes even managing to prise a half-hearted laugh from me.

She started on Barbara's predecessor.

'He was lucky he wasn't sacked, you know. It was this time, three or four years ago.' She paused to check I was still with her. 'He decided to decorate the ward for Christmas.'

'Oh right,' I said.

Ferguson House had a grand name but it was little more than a temporary prefab with high-security doors and windows, bad plumbing and peeling paintwork. It could have done with being spruced up.

'God knows what he was thinking. He put up streamers and tinsel, and then decided to light candles in the corridor.' She laughed. 'Candles in this joint. Can you believe it? With all these arsonists and nutters.'

Clearly another one of us who hadn't completely got to grips with the place.

When Lorraine wasn't around, I had Heather as my named nurse. One day when I was feeling particularly low, she praised Mark.

'You've got a good man there, Helen,' she said.

'I know,' I said.

'Yes,' she said. 'Any other man would have left you.'

32

Late one Thursday morning just after New Year, Craig charged into my room, practically clambering over Amanda, who was on constant outside my door. For once I wasn't sitting on the bed staring out of the window but was in the armchair, listening to David Bowie on my CD player, and reading parasitology research papers. My boss had recently been to visit me and I'd requested some papers from work. I was preparing for the day – as if it was approaching – when I was getting out of there.

'There's someone here to see you,' Craig said. The sycophancy he was spewing was not for my benefit. A man in a dark green woollen overcoat was waiting outside the room.

Craig turned to speak to him. 'Come in,' he said. 'This is Helen Taylor. She's *working*.' I was disappointed he didn't choke on his own contempt.

I didn't get up. The man shook my hand and introduced himself as John Lamb. From then on, whenever I spoke of him, I always referred to him by his full name, but when I was with him I never knew how to address him. Considering the things that I ended up revealing about myself, John was the least of the familiarities, but it felt too intimate to be on first-name terms. On the other hand, Mr Lamb made him sound like a religious studies teacher. In the end, I settled for the cop-out that we'd all resorted to as teenagers with the parents of our friends. As long as I could get away with it, I wouldn't call him anything.

There was only one chair in my room and I didn't offer it. Amanda was keeping an eye through the open door.

'Here, Mr Lamb, take this one. I don't have to hang around.' She flopped her glossy magazine onto the floor and dragged the bulky armchair through the door. He went to help her. I stayed where I was.

Before she left, Amanda said she'd be nearby if she was needed. It almost turned me inside out when I realised the words were meant for me.

John Lamb took off his overcoat, folded it neatly and hung it over the arm of the chair. He settled down. I expected him to take out a pen, paper for clinical notes, a folder to lean on, before pounding me with unwelcome questions. But he did none of those things. He seemed to be waiting for me to start. Reluctantly, I gave in to manners and placed the paper I'd been reading on top of the pile at my feet. We stared at each other. I knew who he was because I'd been told to expect him. John Lamb was the most senior consultant clinical psychologist working in the district. I didn't know if I'd been referred to him because I was so ill or because I was reaping the benefits of medical nepotism. All I knew was that not everyone was afforded the same privileges as me and, for all of our sakes, I wished they hadn't singled me out.

I'd been expecting a younger man. Perhaps hoping for one too, with an eye to resistance or even manipulation. John Lamb didn't look like the sort of person I'd find easy to dupe or to swear at. He was contained, polite and thoroughly incorruptible. That said, it was of no consequence. I wasn't ready for a heart-to-heart.

Weak sunlight trickled into the room between the grimy streaks on the locked-down windows. John Lamb smiled at me and I scowled back. In the background, David Bowie sang songs of darkness and dismay. When I couldn't tolerate the standoff any longer, I got up and, stepping carefully over the papers at my feet, turned the music off.

'What are you reading?'

'Work.' I didn't elaborate.

'I see.'

I saw too. I saw that he was no different from Dr Lorimer. I saw how he was appraising me. I saw how he thought I was kidding myself. How he thought I wasn't going back to work any time soon. But he didn't know me. He didn't know what I was capable of. Just because his corduroy-clad crony had resorted to the underhand tactic of sectioning me didn't mean the fuckers were going to win. But weariness had made my anger flow more slowly and now my animosity seethed below the surface.

We started with a few direct questions. I replied with non-committal grunts. He tried some open-ended questions but I shut them down. He didn't demand answers and I couldn't work out his strategy. For most of the hour, I stared at my bedside cabinet, at the corner where the laminate had started to peel, weighing up the satisfaction of ripping it off like a plaster versus the dissatisfaction of having a cabinet with a sticky, laminate-free wound. Next, I studied my collection of CDs, which I had lined up on the shelf above the built-in cupboard for my clothes. Their spines were organised in rainbow order and the arrangement soothed me. I considered which ones to ask Mark to bring in next and whether to send some home or keep increasing the collection for a wider choice at the risk of spoiling my design. I examined from a distance the Polaroid photos of the cat that I'd stuck above the bed with Blu Tack and looked at the beanie cat, who was lying across my pillow and was a present from my sister, who realised how much I was missing the real one. I wondered what impression of me John Lamb had made from the room alone and preferred not to dwell on it.

From the corridor came the clatter of the dinner trolley pushing through the fire doors and unloading in the kitchen. Raised voices called the lunchtime instructions to staff and patients. In my room, we sat unspeaking. I glanced at John Lamb. He seemed to be meditating. I looked away, grudgingly admiring his capacity to let the silence run.

By the time the first session ended, I had barely said a word. I had also missed lunch. No one had thought to save me anything.

If the therapy sessions were hard going for me, they must have been interminable for John Lamb. He was not excluded from the resentment that I poured over everyone who tried to help me. I was convinced nobody – not even a consultant clinical psychologist – would understand the way I was feeling. Probably because I didn't understand myself.

And yet, when the end of the hour approached, I'd panic. My chance to have someone listen to me, to help me make sense of what was going on, to legitimise my feelings and my situation, had been wasted. He'd leave, with my torment mostly unsaid, and I'd count the hours until the next appointment when I could sit there in silence and churn.

33

One afternoon, there was a commotion.

'Get your filthy pig's hands off me, you fucker.'

It was Sadie being frog-marched back to the ward by a couple of policemen, her tiny frame dwarfed by the two men. As she swore, she spat out strands of her platinum hair that had strayed into her mouth. Her denim jacket was plastered in mud, her t-shirt ripped at the shoulder, exposing her black lacy bra, and her tights laddered. A round of applause broke out among the patients. Sadie had absconded from the hospital for a night and had got shit-faced on cheap vodka and smack. She took a bow. She was a returning heroine. She was my heroine.

Sadie's example put the idea of escape firmly back on my agenda. From then on, whenever an opportunity arose, I pounced on it, attempting to squeeze through the open door as the dinner trolley came in, or following the cleaners as they slipped out the side door. But I was watched all the time. If I was going to abscond for real, make it count, show the doubters that they didn't know shit, I was going to have to up my game.

*

I jumped at the chance of yoga. Not literally, obviously, because my starved, inactive muscles had wasted to scrag ends. The yoga classes were run by a woman who came from the real world. My motivation for signing up was certainly not to work on my sun salutations or my downward dog. The classes took place in the next-door ward, Paterson House, and brought with them the opportunity to step outside.

To get to the class, I was accompanied there and back by whoever was on constant with me. To begin with, my keeper stayed for the duration. After a few classes, they left me to it, and I was taken back to the ward by one of the Paterson nurses. I sussed quite early that there was potential for an inadvertent cock-up.

The yoga level couldn't even be classed as beginner. Most of us were on drugs that affected our balance, our movement and our weight. If we got halfway to touching our toes, that was a bonus. Even lying flat on the mat induced swirling vertigo in me. The class was serenaded by a great deal of farting and groaning, which was both hilarious and repulsive. I didn't let it put me off.

It took some weeks before the opportunity presented itself. In the end-of-class confusion of collecting mats, of thanking the yogi, of putting shoes back on and sorting patients into their respective wards, I slipped out the side door and made a run for it.

The second I was spotted, pandemonium broke out. Shouts and slamming doors. Emergency phone calls. Pursuers on my tail. I made it past Ferguson House. Aiming for the station. Behind me, Laugh-a-Minute Les shouting expletives. I could hear him catching up. I picked up my speed but my wasted legs couldn't keep pace. My desire to flee plunged me forward but the momentum threw me off balance. I went flying, slamming into the pavement face first. My glasses were thrown from my face. I tasted blood. I scrabbled for my specs, scrambled to get to my feet, made it to my knees, but my pursuers were on me within seconds. Les rugby-tackled me back to the ground. I couldn't breathe. Gentle John lumbered up behind, his belly jiggling under his uniform t-shirt. He reached us and trampled straight over my glasses.

'You're hurting me.' My protests were not much louder than a whisper. Everything hurt. My elbows were grazed, my face was bleeding, asphalt shrapnel was wedged under the skin of my palms, my jeans were shredded and I could sense the dull quickening of bruises on my chin, on my knees, on my elbows.

Les sniggered. He grabbed my upper arm and dragged me to my feet.

At last I found my voice. 'Fuck off,' I yelled, squirming under his grip. 'Get off me.' He only tightened his grasp.

Gentle John took the other side of me and the two of them dragged me towards the ward, my toes scuffing the pavement, while I thrashed and writhed under their grip.

'Jesus, I'm coming. Get the fuck off me. John, please. Look, I'm coming. You don't need to—'

But John wouldn't look. The pair of them dragged me up the slope to the front door of Ferguson House.

'I need my glasses. Where are my fucking glasses? Jesus Christ, let me go.'

'Not a fucking chance,' Les said.

'I'm considering IPCU,' Dr Lorimer said. IPCU was the intensive psychiatric care unit. I'd heard about it.

It was the place for the irredeemably mad and the criminally insane.

'Please, no,' I said, fear gripping the back of my neck.

'Last chance. Let's up the diazepam to ten milligrams three times a day.'

If nothing else, it meant that I could hold my own with the patients' conversation in the TV room on the few occasions that I ventured back there.

'Ten milligrams doesnae touch me these days,' someone would say.

'Me neither,' I'd say, and they would look at me in astonishment.

'You speak.'

By six months my hair had grown thin and straggly below my shoulders. Ailsa, an alcoholic in for rehab, was a hairdresser and set herself up in business on the ward, cutting, blow-drying, curling and straightening for customers who sat on the chair beside her bed. The ward tasted of styling mousse and hair lacquer. She shaped my hair into an orderly bob at odds with my appearance. I admired her steady hands. Mine shook constantly – I could barely write or hold a coffee cup. My writing had changed from a flowing italic to a scrawl that looked as if it had been written by a spider on caffeine.

My weight dropped to six and a half stone. Dr Lorimer confronted me with the alternatives.

'We can either carry on as we are, which doesn't seem to be helping, or we can think about electroconvulsive therapy.'

'Fuck off, there's nothing fucking wrong with me.'

I had six lots of ECT and lost my short-term memory.

There was a delicious feeling of losing consciousness as I fought the anaesthetic. Each time, I tried to keep my eyes open and fixed on the operating light, which blurred in and out of focus above me. And each time, I gave in to the drugs and slipped into another world. And when I awoke, I barely knew my own name. It was the first real escape that I had managed.

I saw Davy, the lad who had attacked me, before he left the ward. His eyes no longer flashed with visions he couldn't control. Instead they were glassy and cooperative. He shook my hand.

'I hope you get home soon, doll,' he said.

34

A few months before publication, a lawyer reads my manuscript to check for passages that could be defamatory. It turns out that there are a few things I can't say even if I genuinely believe them to be true, and most of them are from the previous chapter. I make the suggested changes – delete some anecdotes about life on the ward, disguise some characters more than I already have, soften some of my more contentious convictions – and I tie myself in knots trying to stay faithful to the truth. Afterwards, I worry that the revisions might have diminished my story, or worse, that they might not be extensive enough and I'll find myself in trouble. And it makes me question, yet again, the wisdom of writing this book.

35

Things changed. The ECT may have zapped holes in my memory so I lost huge chunks of the recent past, but it definitely flicked a switch. Ferguson House became my home. Not a home I liked, but a home nonetheless. I began to behave almost like a human being. I ate a bit more. I was less agitated. I began to interact with other people in a way that could pass as normal. The cleaner came into my room every morning and we always said hello. I watched the way she looped the hems of the bed-side curtains back on themselves so she could sweep or mop underneath them. I gobbled up these scraps of friendliness and useful household tips.

The memory loss from ECT was weird. It was different from anything I had ever experienced. Years of stress and anxiety had already messed with my memory, I was aware of that, but it was a memory loss that I recognised. A problem of recall. Where did I leave my keys? What day is my next appointment? Oh, I forgot you were coming. There was always a recognition that the memory escaped me, that it was just out of my grasp, that if I tried hard enough I'd be able to trap it. The effect of ECT was dif-ferent. Memories had been swallowed into a black hole and had ceased to exist, and I didn't know what I didn't know. I didn't know if I'd watched certain films, if I'd been to certain places, if I knew certain people. When I was confronted with evidence that I had, it was like witnessing the life of a stranger. It would be something that would come to bother me more when I was out in the real world. In the hospital, it didn't make much odds.

I survived on my routines, on my jigsaws, my books, my music, my visitors. The ECT had dampened my obsession to escape, but thoughts of death were never far from my mind. The catatonic state in which I had found myself at my most severe had shrouded me in many ways, protected me from my excoriating feelings, but now it had passed, I was aware more than ever of how shit I was feeling and how badly I wanted to die. The ECT had led to a superficial improvement in my condition but no one, not even Dr L, could claim it was a miracle cure.

The moment it was decided I could be trusted, it was agreed that Newly Qualified Nicola could take me out.

She came to fetch me from my room. I was lost in *The Mill on the Floss.*

'What are you reading?' she asked.

I showed her the novel.

'Oh, yes. I did George Eliot as part of my degree.'

'Part of your nursing degree?'

'No, don't be daft. English lit.'

The second time she took me out, she told me she was recently married. She said her husband was a lawyer. That they were childhood sweethearts. I told her I thought that was cute.

It was a while before she could take me out again.

When she did, she said she was saving up to go travelling. She was planning to go to Vietnam and Cambodia. If she went to Australia, she might get agency nursing work.

'What about your husband? Can he work there too?'

'What?'

'Your husband?'

'Huh? I'm not married. You thought I was married? That's hilarious.'

'But you . . .'

A few weeks later she told me that she was gay, and I wondered at first if she had pretended to be married because she hadn't come out at work yet. But when I asked her more – about her partner, about her plans, about her English literature degree – she scuttled around my questions. That's when I realised. She was trying out different skins, chameleon-like, blending in or standing out whichever way her fancy took her, practising her masquerade before she went out into the wild. I don't know who her performance was aimed at. It wasn't like she was trying to impress *me*. She didn't give a fuck that I had seen right through her. She didn't even pretend that I had somehow got confused. As far as she was concerned, my opinion of her was worthless.

36

For the entire fourteen months of that first admission, Mark never missed a visit. It is only reading back that I can see how absent he seems at the beginning of my hospital stay. Things had been happening to me and around me, but I had given up all agency over them. As I began to reconnect, Mark became more present. Lunchtime and evening, he'd fuss over me and stay too long. He brought Dorset muesli for my breakfast and mini cartons of orange juice to put on it so I didn't have to have milk. He brought Encona chilli sauce to anaesthetise the taste of the hospital food. And in the evening, he brought apple-pie slices and coffee from the Italian café, and we did the *Herald* cryptic crossword together. However hole-riddled my brain was after the ECT, somehow I could still decipher the clues.

I had hundreds of visitors. Family, friends, work colleagues. My older sister was always there. My parents often. My brother and my younger sister came over from France, where they were both living. My friends came all the time, even though they hated the place, hated seeing me there, seeing me like that. They came even though the chat was stilted because my conversational skills had not recovered and because so many topics seemed off-limits.

They came even though they all had other crap going on in their lives. And if they couldn't come, they sent cards and letters to let me know that I was always in their thoughts.

My room was constantly bedecked with flowers. Keeping them healthy became one of the few tasks I was invested in. At the sink in my room, I filled the plastic water jug I used as a vase and arranged the bouquets. To keep the flowers healthy, I cleaned the jug and changed the water regularly. To refresh the stems, I had to ask for scissors from the supplies in the treatment room. I was allowed surgical scissors with two-centimetre blades to trim the stalks. And I was to make sure I always handed them back.

It was during these months that two patients, Coleen and Gail, befriended me on one of the rare times I bothered to queue at the canteen. Friday was fish and chip day, and the chips were the only thing I found even partially edible. They sat down at the same table as me, unaware that they were battering down the invisible barriers that I had constructed to protect myself. They asked my name. How long I'd been in. What I was in for. I told them depression. They seemed surprised, said that they thought I had anorexia. It felt churlish to point out that I had, but not in the way they meant, that the medical term for not eating was the same no matter what the underlying cause. As with Lorraine, I felt like they were mothering me, although I was certain they were no older than I was. With unashamed candour, they told me a little of their circumstances, their mental health issues, their drug use, their stories of abuse and violent relationships. They told me where they lived and I knew it from its reputation. They talked about their kids and their fights with social workers and their last chances to keep them. And once again, I cringed with shame at what a piece of piss my life was.

One day Gail came back on a high after meeting with her consultant. We were drinking weak tea in the dining room.

She gave Coleen the thumbs-up. 'Mood stabilisers,' she said.

'You lucky bitch,' Coleen said. 'They said I couldn't have them.'

'That's ridiculous. Honestly, they should give them to everyone. What about you, H?'

Mood stabilisers? I had no idea what they were talking about. I might have been medically trained, but they were far more informed than I was.

'You should ask for them. No joke, hen, they are fucking miracle drugs,' Coleen said. 'Who's your consultant?'

Sadly, it transpired that mood stabilisers included the lithium that I was already on. It seemed that once again I would have to wait for a miracle cure.

As the months passed, I was allowed more time out of the ward. After lunch, Mark would take me to a greasy-spoon café around the corner from the hospital. The café was a halfway house, the first step back to the outside world for many of us, and most of the clientele were familiar from the ward. Mark and I took the back lane to it, picking our way between the puddles on the unsurfaced alleyway, and marking the passing of the seasons by the changing foliage and whatever blooms were in the flowerpots on the back stairs of the two-storey flats. The coffee was terrible, as insipid and thin as the coffee on the ward, but we sweetened it by eating Tunnock's wafers alongside. To this day, they still taste of freedom.

'You off out, doll?' Billy said, breaking away from the smoking huddle one afternoon.

'Yes,' I said. This was not the type of conversation that I usually had with Billy. The type that involved obscenities and spitting and aggressive psychosis, and which scared the pants off me.

'Right.' He stood beside me, staring at the road while he finished his fag. I shifted from one foot to the other, waiting for the aggro to start.

A few minutes later Mark pulled up outside the ward in our Micra. He waved to me as he got out of the car.

'That your car?'

'Yes,' I said.

'Aye? Well, it's a fucking wee car for youse two lanky bastards.'

Couldn't really argue with that.

37

'I feel for you, Helen. I understand. Really.'

We were outside in what passed for summer. I was with my friend Danny. We were doing loops of the hospital grounds, around the psych wards and up to the general hospital. I was working on an alternative escape plan that involved rebuilding my muscle strength and a legitimate discharge. I'd recently started physiotherapy sessions up in the old building for precisely that reason. Whenever I could, I attended physio three or four times a week. The physiotherapist started me on gentle mat work before she let me loose on the proper equipment. After a couple of sessions getting used to the rowing machine and the cross-trainer, she gave me a fitness programme and left me to manage it myself. It was strange being back in a gym. I'd been a member of the university one and had used it regularly, testing my speed and endurance and strength in an unspoken competition with the staff or students on the neighbouring machines.

In the hospital gym, I frequently shared the space with a couple of blokes from the outpatient AA group. They'd huff and puff on the cross-trainer and the rowing machine, and wheeze and stomp on the treadmill while I did my thing. When my turn came to give the treadmill a go, the physio suggested taking it slowly to allow for my unsteady gait – a consequence of all the meds I was on – and my general poor fitness. But my competitive streak hadn't wasted as quickly as my muscles. When the telephone called the physio to her office, I took my chance to up the speed from walking pace to a gentle jog. It felt good. I wanted to show the AA guys that this was just a warm-up. I edged it up further. Excitement buzzed through me as my legs were stretched and tested. The failed escape after yoga class was long behind me and my legs felt stronger. I turned the speed up further, keeping my finger on the button. The digital speedometer skipped up several kilometres per hour. I started to run. But the response delay of the treadmill caught me out. Within seconds, the mat was turning too fast. I was being dragged away from the controls, barely able to keep up. My feet were slapping the running mat, my legs were frantic, my arms flailing to keep balance. In desperation, I lunged for the dial but didn't make it. I whizzed backwards off the treadmill and landed in a heap. One of the men rushed over and helped me to my feet.

'The thing is, hen,' he said, 'you've gottae stay off the sauce.'

Now I was taking it more steadily, building up strength and stamina both on the treadmill and with regular walks. Every visitor was commandeered to take me out, whatever the weather.

'Look at that,' I said to Danny. In a doorway at the back of a medical ward where I'd done a placement as a student, a couple of patients and their visitors were smoking. One of the patients had an oxygen tank.

'Don't get too near,' I said. 'We could go up with the blast.'

Danny glanced over. Despite the threat, he ignored them and continued empathising. 'The thing is, we've all been there.'

I smiled blandly, as much as the max-strength diazepam I gobbled three times a day would allow me. It bugged me that those patients were allowed to get away with killing themselves slowly (although it was true that the oxygen tank added an element of unpredictability and potential haste to their eventual demise) and that their behaviour was facilitated by their visitors, while all my treatment was focused on preventing me doing an accelerated version of the same thing. And without putting other people at risk. But my anger smouldered now instead of flared. I was probably easier to deal with, but even I found myself boring. Anyway, I didn't want to be mad at Danny. I was glad of the company and glad of his concern and I didn't have the energy to contradict him. But he was wrong. He had to be wrong. It wasn't possible that everyone had been where I had been, where I still was. Because if that was the case, why was I in hospital when everyone else was valiantly getting on with whatever life chucked at them?

Danny had stuck his nail in an ulcer of my own making. Constant niggling, poking, picking and worrying had made it worse as I worked my way towards discharge. I was forever turning to Lorraine to put a sticking plaster over it, but she wouldn't always be there. Anyway, I was sick of my dependency, sick of seeking validation that I was actually ill. I had conned everyone, Dr L, Lorraine, John Lamb. Danny was right. Everyone knew what it was like to feel depressed. I was wallowing. Depression, or at least my version of it, wasn't a legitimate illness. Not like schizophrenia or bipolar disorder. They were proper illnesses with clear symptoms that your average man or woman on the street would be unlikely to have experienced. They were the stuff of films and classic literature, unusual and distinct enough to merit special record: visual hallucinations, auditory hallucinations, florid delusions. In many ways I was envious. To suffer like that must be totally shit but at least the whole world and his granny couldn't claim that they knew how it was to be afflicted. I didn't believe I was John the Baptist or Queen Elizabeth I. I didn't have imaginary friends like Davy or voices telling me to piss in the shower. The radio didn't send me coded messages and the people in the television didn't come out and visit me at night. Those patients were suffering through no fault of their own. Their symptoms were not a result of lack of willpower or inherent weakness. They were unlucky. They deserved help. I didn't deserve help. I was just, well, a bit depressed.

It didn't matter that I had severe paranoia and delusions of a different type, or that I had intrusive thoughts and a persistent, nagging internal monologue telling me how crap I was at everything and that I should just end it, and another scornful and determined that I shouldn't be allowed to get off so lightly. I was a fraud and an imposter. Like Danny said, I couldn't even do depression properly.

We carried on up the hill in silence, through the car park, towards the swan pond. An old woman, wrapped in several scarves and an overcoat far too warm for even the pallid attempt at summer, was sitting on one of the park benches throwing morsels of bread to screeching gulls who circled and jostled in the air above her. At the other side of the pond, the swans glided among the weed and bobbing lager cans with their adolescent cygnets following their haughty example. They thought themselves too good for their surroundings. A gust of wind rippled the pond and sent the gulls reeling. The woman cooed to them. I shivered and wondered what loneliness had brought her there.

Back on the ward, as discharge approached, the changes accelerated around me. Stepped decreases in observations, more time out, trials at home. I should have been grateful that my plan was coming together, but I was crippled by a deep terror of what lay ahead without the protection of the ward.

Scott recognised my fear and did his best to soothe it. He was a lovely man. Even though his job as a nursing assistant was secondary to his dreams for rock-and-roll stardom, he was a natural at it. He had a rare honesty. He was honest in his regard for me. Honest in his motivation and his aspirations. At times, his honesty scarred him like a branding iron and it was raw and ugly. One afternoon, not that long before my formal discharge, he came to see me, flustered and upset. A local band he knew had signed a record deal. He was reeling from the injustice.

'Can you believe it?' he said. 'They were our flipping support act. Now they reckon they're the big shots.'

He couldn't hide the pain of his envy. A pain that wasn't eased when the band went on to have major, mainstream success. To make Scott feel better, we agreed they had sold out.

38

Home. Without the structure of the hospital day, I was floundering. Geraldine, the community psychiatric nurse assigned to me at discharge, encouraged me to make a list of daily tasks and tick them off so that I could see I had achieved something.

'Small steps,' she said, and kept repeating.

My task list read much like the diary I had kept when I was seven.

Get up.

Have breakfast.

It was rarely more ambitious than that.

I don't remember when Mark first dared go back to work. There must have been a gradual letting-go as I was passed between services. After hospital, my medical care was taken over by the intensive community therapy unit, or ICT as it was known, where I had regular appointments and which was open for drop-ins in case of emergency. Whenever I had to leave the house to attend, I went by taxi. I wasn't capable of making the journey under my own steam. Geraldine helped me fill out forms for DLA – Disability Living Allowance – and other benefits. She said they were meant for exactly those type of expenses. I said they were meant for folk who were struggling, not for folk who lived in neighbourhoods where most people parked their BMWs in their double garages. Frankly, I had to get off my arse, stop dossing around and get back to work. Except that, for the moment, I could barely get out of bed. When guilt and anxiety had me climbing the walls, Geraldine talked me down. Her refrain seldom changed: *If you had had cancer, you wouldn't put so much pressure on yourself.* But I hadn't had cancer. I hadn't had so much as a common cold. And it wasn't like we were skint. I shouldn't be getting paid for pissing about. Not only was I a burden to my family, I'd become a burden to the state. I wanted to send my benefit to my comrades from the ward. At least they could have used it to brighten up their days. DLA or, as we liked to call it, Drugs and Lager Allowance.

Wrong, in so many ways.

My consultant at ICT was Dr Hargreaves. She was at a disadvantage from the off. It had taken fourteen months of putting Dr L through hell before I'd accepted that he'd had my best interests at heart. I wasn't about to change my loyalty overnight. Mark tells me I liked her at the time. That's not how I remember it. Perhaps my opinion has been twisted by what was to come. An offhand remark that shattered my opinion of her. But you must tread carefully with the paranoid and the persecuted.

Either way, I missed Dr Lorimer. We had come to understand each other. Or, at least, that's how I saw it. I suspect that he was glad to see the back of me. He had practically told me as much when I left Ferguson House, making it clear that he wasn't at all keen to welcome me there again. An attitude that I found surprisingly inhospitable, given how well we'd got to know each other.

'I don't get how all this talking is meant to change how I feel,' I said to John Lamb at one of our regular Tuesday afternoon appointments. Which was kind of ironic, as I had barely muttered a word during the previous forty minutes. I'd spent most of the session staring out of the first-floor window, studying the way the downpipe connected to the gutter of the porch roof and contemplating the potential satisfaction to be derived from scraping the pillows of moss off the roof tiles. John Lamb was sitting in his armchair on the far side of the bay window and had apparently zoned out. His eyes flickered open when I spoke.

'How's it supposed to work?' I said. 'Am I supposed to keep talking until I miraculously feel better?' It made no sense to me at all. If it was simply to reach an understanding of how fucked-up my thought patterns were, we were time-wasting on an epic scale. It wasn't that I didn't understand my perverse thinking. I just didn't know how to make it stop.

John Lamb gave a wry smile. He quoted hypotheses and studies and theories.

I scoffed.

If I didn't have an appointment to force me to get up in the morning, I rarely completed even the first of my daily tasks. Generally, I'd loll around in bed, watching the daylight trace its path across the curtainless windows and listening to the magpies squabbling in the trees behind the house, or to the thrum of municipal gardeners mowing the playing fields or strimming the verge, or to trains rattling their way into town, until I'd succeeded in murdering the best part of the day. If the phone rang, I ignored it. Likewise, the doorbell. Jehovah's Witnesses aside, my only unscheduled visitors were the window cleaners, who buzzed the door before they started, to give me fair warning to get my cash ready. Whatever the time of day – usually late morning or early afternoon – I refused to answer. At the sound of the clattering ladders, the cat would panic and hide under the bed. I'd pull the duvet over my head and pretend to be asleep. Even though they could spy me as they sponged and shammied the casement window, my sloth-like behaviour meant they were forced to put a note through the door asking for the money. It must have driven them crazy to see the lump of me curled up under the covers. I bet they thought I was too tight to pay.

My days might have been spent loafing around in bed, but it didn't mean I was well rested. My nights were shattered by insomnia. It was frenetic. Waking dreams where a thousand electronic screens would flash and strobe before my eyes. Where there were voices distorted by static, faces I had no time to focus on, and a frenzy of disapproval and disgust that I could only feel. And all of them jabbering and jeering and all of them wanting a piece of me.

On the edge of sleep, I would jolt awake, electrocuted by a rogue cable. Awake, I would shut my eyes but couldn't extinguish the power supply.

I became impossible to live with. Without the mind-numbing tedium of the ward, there was nothing to dampen the noise in my head. The battle between the bullies who tormented my nightmares was unleashed in daylight. There were those who taunted me for how useless I was, how worthless, that my life wasn't worth living, and those that said I was weak and pathetic and didn't deserve to die. It was incessant. Like the pain of a migraine, I couldn't see beyond it. Couldn't even see around the edges. I was blinkered by my desperation to silence them. I turned my sight inwards. Directed all of my focus towards making it stop.

39

'For fuck's sake. What did you do that for?'

'I didn't do anything.'

'You crept up on me. You made me jump. You know what I'm like.'

'It doesn't matter,' Mark said, after he'd denied the creeping.

But it did matter. I'd smashed my favourite mug. Whacked it off the corner of the work surface. It had cracked and smashed on the kitchen floor. I'd been left holding the broken handle.

Mark had bought me the mug from Tate Modern the first time we'd gone, not long after its conversion from Bankside power station, when we'd seen the magnificence of Louise Bourgeois' *Maman*, the gigantesque spider mother which was, at once, astonishingly beautiful and utterly repellent. A marble egg sac hung from her underside as a symbol of both her absolute power and her desperate vulnerability, and meant that even in that moment of high art, it was impossible for me to escape a life dominated by cycles, hormones, follicles and eggs. The mug had survived the taint of London-water tea stains in our Crouch End flat, it had survived a round of duty as a coffee mug in the Mill Hill lab at the Research Institute, and it had survived a house move to Scotland. But it hadn't survived the jitters that twanged my nerves like catgut.

MO, DER, N and some pieces like extracted teeth.

I hadn't consciously invested a value in that particular mug before it was broken, but in pieces it represented everything that was of any importance: our London life, those months of snatched happiness and hope, us.

I stooped to pick up the lettered fragments.

'Leave it, Helen,' Mark said. 'Leave it. I'll do it. I'll get the hoover.'

I ignored him and picked at the fragments, cupping the larger pieces in my hands and reassembling them into a mug shape. I was good at this. I'd had practice. There was, after all, a reason for doing those hospital jigsaws.

'Have we got superglue?'

Mark laughed. 'I think it's slightly beyond repair.'

'I want to stick it together.' He didn't realise. He simply didn't. It wasn't the mug I was sticking together.

'We can get another one.'

'Like when? When can we get another one?'

'I meant . . . Give it here.' He reached for the broken pieces. I snatched them away. 'Come on, Helen.'

'No. I'll do it.' It was pointless. It was in bits. My life, our life, was in bits.

'Let me—'

'I'll do it. I'm not useless. You think I'm useless.' I was yelling now, crushing the broken fragments in my fist. Ramming a jagged edge into my fingers.

'Leave it. You'll hurt yourself.'

But I already had. A bead of blood quivered on my middle finger. I sucked it. It tasted of battery acid.

'See. You're bleeding.'

'Go on, then. You do it. You're right. I can't do anything. I'm a fucking waste of space.' I threw the broken fragments across the floor.

Just to spite me, Mark refused to get riled. He went to get the dustpan from under the sink.

'Fuck. The fuck. Off,' I spat. The words smacked off the kitchen walls but he didn't react. His back as he squatted to reach into the cupboard under the sink was unruffled. His shoulders were steady as he reached behind the box of dishwasher tablets and the spare pack of pan scourers. I was incensed. Beside myself with rage. And livid that he had done nothing to deserve my fury. Except, of course, connive to tether me to life.

I watched him unfold himself with the dustpan and brush in his hand. He looked at me with a weariness in his eyes that I hadn't seen before. My anger chilled with the hiss of lava hitting the sea. Basalt set in my veins. He'd had enough, I could tell. I couldn't blame him. It had to stop. Once and for all.

My chance was right there. Blades wedged in the knife block. I snatched a carving knife and fled the kitchen, hacking at my wrist as I ran, too haphazardly to break the skin. At my heels, the plastic clatter of dustpan and brush. Straight off, Mark was on to me. He read my moves. Blocked my escape. Blocked the front door. Barred the stairs. Backed me into a corner in the hall. I was trapped under the coat pegs. Smothered by winter coats. Barricaded by a tumbling pyramid of old shoes. My chance was slipping away. The smell of musty wool and stale insoles threatened to stifle me. I kicked the shoes out of the way, shoved the coats out of my face. Mark was yelling at me to put the knife down, to not be so stupid; if I didn't care about myself, at least to think about him. And I was yelling back, telling him to keep away from me, that it was my choice, my right, that it was better for everyone, and I was waving the knife around, near my neck, my wrists, slashing at the coats, wildly jabbing the blade towards him as he tried to stop me, wondering which one of us I was going to kill. He lunged at me, made a grab for the knife, but I ducked and fled back into the kitchen. I was at the back door, jiggling the key, desperately turning the lock. Mark grabbed me from behind and pinned my arms to my sides. We'd stopped yelling. We were both panting, our struggle punctuated by gasps. Mark wrested the knife from my grip and flung it towards the wall cabinets. It landed on the top of a cupboard and slid behind. For a second, we paused. Waited for the knife to reappear. A cartoon moment. Off the cliff. Still running without falling. But the knife was stuck, jammed between the cabinet and the uneven plaster.

Mark's grip loosened an instant and I dived for the knife block, for the rest of the knives. But he was fast. Faster. He grabbed the block. Slammed it in a cupboard. Stood guard against the door. I pummelled him with my fists, howling. He let me hit him, only raising his arms to shield the worst of my blows. When I had spent the last of my rage, I collapsed. Slumped to my hands and knees, dripping tears and snot onto the floor, shuddering with ugly gulps while a separate part of me watched the drops spatter and noticed the pattern of sticky asterisks they formed on the lino tiles. Mark knelt beside me and put his arms around me. I sank into him.

From then on, all the knives were hidden or locked

away. We bought sliced bread for toast and ate a lot of ready meals. The lost knife had been part of a wedding-present set. Later, when we moved, we would consider taking the cupboard off the wall to reunite the missing member with its surviving companions but instead we left the memory hidden. Turns out Mark hid a whole pile of knives behind the same cupboard. Or so he tells me now. I wonder if the new owners ever found them.

Our days weren't always so traumatic. Interludes of peace were scattered among them. I took lorazepam for anxiety flares and sleeping tablets for insomnia. Because I'd been off alcohol for a year and a half in hospital, a single glass of wine would get me tipsy. Saturday nights became fizz nights. We bought half bottles of champagne from M&S and drank them watching *The X Factor* or some other crap on the TV, me in my tartan PJs with the cat on my knee stealing crisps out of my hand. We snatched these moments of respite. But I was afraid of the surge of love for them both that surfaced with the bubbles.

Mark did everything for me. The supermarket shopping, the driving, the cooking. We joked about his limited repertoire but, even without knives to prepare it, compared to the ward, the food was *MasterChef* quality. Yet I took no pleasure in it. I stressed over gaining weight because my thinness had become the physical manifestation – the irrefutable proof – of my illness. If I gained weight, I wouldn't be so gaunt. I wouldn't look unwell. And if I didn't look unwell, then I'd be judged by others the way I judged myself. Geraldine insisted I be kind to myself. She envisaged bubble baths and scented candles and relaxation CDs.

But I couldn't bring myself to imagine even my own idea of kindness. So Mark did it for me. He bought me music, printed out hundreds of photos of the cat. He employed a cleaner, and a lad to keep the worst of the garden under control. I kept expecting him to snap under the pressure of it, under the pressure of me, but, somehow, he kept going. At one point I even accused him of being emotionally bereft. But he wasn't. It was just his way of coping.

It freaked me out at times how narrow our life had become. Not for my sake but for Mark's. Occasionally I agreed to make a trip to the West End of Glasgow, daring only the cafés where we were regulars, where we'd been through the double-takes and the pitying looks, where I didn't have to explain my tremor and my unprovoked despair. Sometimes I looked outside of myself at the pathetic, trembling, dependent creature I had become and wondered how I had ever worked, ever held any position of responsibility, ever considered myself a grown-up. How I had ever thought I could be a parent. And all the time, Heather's words on a feedback loop in my head: *Any other man would have left you.*

On Saturdays we made our weekly trip to the pharmacy to collect my rationed meds because I couldn't be trusted with a full prescription. This drug rationing was another way I was being controlled. Another way I was being infantilised. Recently, the law had changed so that a hospital section was converted to a community treatment order when the patient went home. Insomnia aside, I might have been sleeping in my own bed, but I wasn't at liberty to do what I wanted.

What I wanted, of course, was to kill myself.

40

Imagine this. A rocky plain dotted with cacti, scrub and wild herbs. A desolate place where the daily struggle for survival has you scavenging for roots to nibble and searching for water from streams that have dried to a trickle. Or it would if you weren't constantly waylaid from the task by the wild beasties who inhabit the place, savage wee buggers who totally have it in for you. Your best friend and true companion flies at your shoulder, a willow warbler, as chirpy and lively with her chatter and trills as she is innocuous and unobtrusive in appearance. She sings to keep your spirits up when they are flagging. To be honest, it can get annoying at times.

Life wasn't always like this. Once upon a time, this was a green and pleasant land, a land where, should the fancy take you, you could skip barefoot through luscious grass and bathe in babbling brooks. In the old days, even the beasties were relatively harmless, fluffy and chubby like miniature emus who might take an occasional snap at your ankles at the very worst. But with the passage of time, it is not just the landscape that has hardened. An ankle here, a buttock there, it didn't take long for those nippy wee rascals to become addicted to the taste of your flesh. With each nibbled morsel they morphed into the vicious little shites they are today. Their downy feathers have turned to spiky quills and they are Velociraptor-like, jittery and vindictive with lashing tongues, sharp teeth, raptor claws. And they are ravenous for you. Your daily trek across this plain with Willow fluttering above you is becoming increasingly hazardous. She is quick enough on the wing to evade their gnashing teeth. You, on the other hand, are easy prey. The attacks have left you injured. You stagger on while they tear out your hair, shred your skin, rip your flesh. Your ear hangs loose and your entrails spill down your front. You don't know how much more you can withstand. Willow tends your wounds with poultices from the herbs she has gathered in her beak, but the wounds don't heal overnight the way they used to.

Someone else walks this land too. It is Johnny Cash from the cover of his first *American Recordings* album. Weirdly, his weapon is not Death's usual scythe, but a rifle from one of his cowboy songs. He watches your feeble attempts to shield yourself from the unrelenting attacks, your futile effort to prise the crazy fuckers off you. He is playing it cool. Giving you space to fight your own battles. You get mad at him for gawping. Yell at him for not coming to your aid. One of the wee bastards has bitten off your finger. Another has gouged a chunk out of your thigh. You have already lost an eye. Before long there will be nothing left of you.

'For fuck's sake!' you screech. One of the creatures has got you around the neck and is going for your jugular. 'Can you not help a body out here?'

In true cowboy style, Johnny slings his rifle from his shoulder. Contemplates the beast with its teeth in your neck. He, as the song goes, draws a bead on it to practise his aim. 'Say the word,' he drawls, 'and I'll fire.'

'The word,' you say, finding yourself vaguely amusing even in your compromised state. But Johnny doesn't fire because he is busy spelling out the conditions of the contract. If he shoots, he explains, you must walk with him, walk beside him, for now and for evermore. He needs an audience to test out his new material. You consider the offer. Although you are mad at him, it doesn't feel too bad to hang out for the rest of time with Johnny Cash. Not when you consider the alternative. Willow flutters over your head. You cannot see her because you can't actually look up, thanks to the fucker guzzling your neck blood, but you know she is there. You can feel the beat of her wings. Hear the lament of her song. If you leave with Johnny, you will miss her. You know she will miss you too, but at least you can spare her the ordeal of having to witness you being mutilated bite by spiteful bite. It isn't ideal, but frankly, it's a no-brainer. You signal to Johnny. He nods. You wish he would just get on with it.

'Shoot, damn it.'

This isn't suicide for the sake of killing yourself. This is suicide as self-preservation.

Of course, it makes no flipping sense. But how else am I supposed to explain it?

41

'Let's try something. I want you to focus on a single moment recently when you felt good.' Geraldine caught the look on my face. 'OK, not good, then. Less bad.'

I scoffed, but she persisted.

'Come on. You must have something.'

'Sunday mornings,' I said, at last.

'Which Sunday morning?'

'Just generally.'

'Doing what?'

'Lying in bed.'

'OK. Close your eyes. What can you see? What can you hear?'

'Mark's reading the paper. I can hear him turning the pages next to me. Every now and then, he reads a bit out, or shows me the fashion in the magazine.'

'Go on.'

'The windows are open. I can hear shouts from the footballers training on the playing fields and the noise of kids playing on the swings. You know, cries of glee. The cat is sat on my chest, rubbing her face into my fingers.' The memory made me smile. I felt wistful. 'I stroke and scratch her cheeks, under her chin, and her lips pucker like she's pouting.' I heard the crack in my voice. Even my version of happiness threatened to be drowned by tears. 'Sometimes she rams her face underneath my chin and nuzzles into my neck. She might stay like that for ages.'

'Go on.'

'She dribbles.'

'Oh.'

I opened my eyes. 'No, no, it's cute. She gets so carried away purring. I can feel her dribble dripping onto my neck. Mark thinks it's minging but it's really, really cute.' I was kind of laughing but my eyes were brimming.

'That feeling,' Geraldine said. 'Guard that feeling.'

But I couldn't guard that feeling. From time to time I tried, but it slipped between my fingers.

42

Time moved on. Christmas, with all its connotations, came and went. By increments, things changed. Almost imperceptibly, my boundaries expanded. First the local shops, then the nearby woods and duck pond. Then other places in the West End, visits to friends nearby, across to the south side to see my in-laws.

It was hard. Too hard at times.

ICT and the psychology unit where John Lamb worked were housed in neighbouring villas on Great Western Road. They were dark sandstone, Victorian, with elaborate cornicing and servants' entrances. I assumed there must have been a fashion for wealthy old women to gift property to the council in their will, keeping up with the Joneses even after death, because it seemed the most rational explanation for why two neighbouring houses were reduced to such circumstances. Or maybe the widows had sold them at a knock-down price when the upkeep for the complicated roofs and fancy stonework had become too pricey. Many similar houses had been divided into flats for precisely those reasons, twenty or thirty years previously. In some pockets, the money was bulging again.

Bankers, lawyers, celebrities were buying up the flats, restoring the properties to their former grandeur (with or without the live-in servants). But for these two, the gardens had been tarmacked over for parking and the doors fitted with security intercoms. I often wondered what the neighbours thought of the clientele. Thanks to the massive NHS signs out front, there was no disguising who we were.

From the outside, the buildings looked grand, but inside they were not immune to institutional squalor: cheap furniture, temperamental window blinds and polystyrene ceiling tiles. In the waiting area, I'd pour myself a cup of plastic water from the cooler and ignore the spread of magazines from three years earlier. To dodge my intrusive thoughts, I'd study the place minutely, even though I was already overly familiar with it. The waiting area was in an entrance hall that had once been magnificent but – divided at intervals by fire doors and decorated with safety signs and fire extinguishers – it had squandered its splendour. Likewise the stairs. Barely any trace of the pattern of the wrought-iron banisters that swept the curve of them remained, definition blunted beneath decades of gloss paint. And the air hung with the musty odour of carpet squares cut with cheap air freshener and antiseptic. For me it was – still is – the smell of dread.

Although I came to detest the visits to ICT, the visits next door to John Lamb were my lifeline. He tolerated my hours of silence, my sullenness, my occasional outbursts. And my tissue-boxes of tears.

Months passed and I began to make my own way there by train. On the station platform, I kept my head down, studiously avoiding eye contact with fellow passengers, staring inwards at the confusion in my brain, terrified I might meet someone I knew. Even now, when I see dandelions shooting up between train tracks, or smell that mix of steel, diesel engines and wet nettles, echoes of that throat-clenching anxiety send me hurtling back there. When the train pulled in to the stop, I'd take the slope down from the station, turn into the main road and trudge past the Art Deco flats which edged the hospital grounds, all the while feeling the presence – the threat – of Ferguson House in the near distance. Out of sight but still exerting its hold.

43

'Did I ever tell you about my transvestite husband, hen?' Sandra asked, placing some tobacco neatly into a cigarette paper.

I spluttered on my coffee. We were sitting outside by the back door, under an overcast sky. I was on the step and Sandra was perched against the garden wall, using the wheelie bin as a coffee table.

'Er, no, I'm pretty sure I would have remembered that,' I said. My memory wasn't quite what it should have been after the ECT, so I could never be entirely sure. I sipped my drink, trying to steady the mug with drug-shaky hands.

Sandra rolled the cigarette with deft fingers. As usual, the colour of her fingernails matched the tips of her spiky hair. Today, they were navy blue. Every Friday, she rocketed around my house, leaving a scorched trail of scrubbed surfaces and vacuumed carpets and an afterburn of bleach fumes before she moved on to do the same elsewhere, and yet her fingernails were always perfectly manicured. I could never figure it out. She wore yellow Marigolds, but even so.

I had come to depend on her. Not just because I was so feeble that I could barely make a bed or fold a tea towel but because Sandra was one of the few people who spoke to me as if I wasn't a freak. We'd pass half of her time gossiping. I'd forgotten what it was like to hold a sane conversation. Although, to be truthful, not many of the conversations we had could properly be described as sane.

'He wasn't the one that kidnapped my boy,' she explained, licking the edge of the cigarette paper. I knew that story. She'd told me it a couple of weeks earlier. After she split from her first husband, she came back to Glasgow with her son, who was about nine at the time, and got a job in a pub in Govan. One summer's evening, when Sandra was at work, husband number one had bundled Jamie into his car and taken him back to London. Fortunately for Sandra, the police tracked them down without difficulty. Unfortunately for Sandra, when she saw her ex-husband in Kilburn police station, she went berserk, calling him every insult in her extensive repertoire and catching him with a practised left hook. Which almost got her arrested. Sandra didn't see her first husband again for years. Then one evening she served him in the pub in Govan without recognising him. 'He'd got fat and bald,' she told me with relish.

She shielded her lighter from the breeze and lit her cigarette. 'This one was a big, violent fucker,' she said, talking about husband number two. Between drags, she told me where he was from. The area was infamous. Drug gangs and loan sharks. Burnt-out Ford Fiestas in the streets and syringes in the play parks. I couldn't imagine that it was a safe place for a man to openly express his feminine side. 'He drove trucks,' she added.

I had in my mind a picture of a broad-shouldered, tattooed trucker with a skinhead. 'So, did he go out dressed up?' I asked, doing my best to picture the transformation. I had so many questions. It felt risqué and slightly exotic.

'Oh no, he only ever dressed up in the house,' Sandra said. 'He used to wear my bra and knickers.'

'But . . .' In my head, I was computing the size discrepancy. Sandra was tiny. Sparrow-thin. Weighed down only by her stack-heeled boots or the chunky slippers that she wore in the house. Beside her, I was an ungainly, lumbering giant.

'Yeah, I know. He stretched the whole lot out of shape. I wouldn't have minded,' she said, 'but it was always my good Marks and Spencer things, never the cheap Primark stuff.'

'What happened to him?'

'I left him after he put me in hospital.'

My interest in him evaporated. I glanced at Sandra to gauge her reaction to what she had just told me, but her emotions were hidden behind a puff of smoke.

'Bloody hell, Sandra, what did he do?'

'Oh, you know. The usual.'

We sat in silence for a few moments. I examined the rip in the knee of my jeans and pulled my sweatshirt sleeves down over my hands. I was so ashamed. Ashamed of my cushy life. Ashamed of the weakness of my depression. Ashamed of the pathetic reasons behind my desperation to kill myself. Ashamed that someone else was cleaning my house for me. Sandra took shallow draws on her roll-up, intermittently flicking the ash into the Coke tin she was using as an ashtray. She opened a packet sandwich that she'd brought for her lunch, and started feeding chunks of it to the cat, who had wandered over from underneath a heather bush. Suddenly she started to laugh, a laugh tinged with tobacco smoke that made her cough.

'When we first met, we'd go out dressed really smart.

He'd wear a suit and a tie. Folk in the pub thought we were CID'.

It figured. The only people you saw wearing a tie in a pub in Govan were plain-clothes detectives. They may as well have worn a sign round their necks.

'He was CID all right.' She paused. 'CID, a cunt in drag.'

44

I spent a lot of time crying. But it wasn't only self-pity and shame that made me weep. It was everything.

Behind our house there was a tiny wood and occasionally deer would stray into our garden. Their skittish presence was magical but their vulnerability made me cry. In spring, our garden burst with daffodils, primroses and delicate snake's-head fritillaries. I recognised their ephemeral beauty, but it also made me cry. We had catmint growing in a plant pot up the back and the cat would rub her face in the leaves, chirrup and squeeze herself into the pot so her flanks bulged over the edges and the plant beneath her was flattened. Her catnip bliss, the simplicity of a life fulfilled by chicken biscuits and plentiful naps, her squishy tummy: other things that made me cry.

'Let's get the hammock out,' Mark suggested one rare, beautiful Sunday morning in early May when we were eating breakfast outdoors. We'd had the hammock since we'd been married – a wedding present, like the hidden knives – but our London garden hadn't had trees strong enough to support it. It was in the garage, wrapped in bin bags tied with parcel tape. Mark went to fetch it. He unfurled it on the grass to examine it. Miraculously, given how damp the flat had been, it had survived in its bin bags without catching mildew.

'Ta-dah,' Mark said, once he'd lashed it between a budding oak and the acer. 'Do you want to give it a go?'

'You first,' I said. He had never been a Boy Scout, my husband. I didn't trust his knot-tying skills.

As he clambered on, the hammock swung and shoogled wildly underneath him, but he steadied it and rearranged himself, stretching out and folding his arms behind his head in a parody of a country bumpkin. I wanted to give him a stalk of grass to chew but he suffered badly from hay fever, and one summer in London I had almost killed him by making him picnic in the long grass on Hampstead Heath. Now, he swung gently in the hammock, assuring me that it was great once you got used to it.

'Yeah?' I should have known better. I could barely keep upright shuffling along on the flat. I was taking my life in my hands climbing into a flimsy bit of cloth floating between the branches of two trees.

'I can't do it,' I said after I'd tried to launch myself first from one side and then the other. The drug shakes, the vertigo, the terror-seized muscles.

'Course you can,' Mark said. 'I'll give you a leg up.'

He knelt down, hands cupped together, and I tentatively put a foot between them. Fine tremors turned to earthquakes. My entire body convulsed.

'One, two, three.'

'Wait!'

Too late. Mark hoiked me up. I flopped onto the hammock, stomach first, felt the sacking twist and give beneath me as I struggled to align myself, and promptly toppled off the other side. I hit the grass with a thud. Mark started to laugh. I tried to stand but I was on a slope. I lost balance before I'd even got off my knees.

'Shit, fuck, shit, shit.' I struck the ground with my right shoulder. Couldn't stop. Tumbled down the grass and onto the steep path. Thuds and bruises marked my descent. Mark tried to grab me but I had too much momentum. I somersaulted down the gravel-shot steps. Saw iris stems on the march. Glimpsed an advancing fence post. Covered my head with my arms just before I hammered into it. For a moment, I lay in the flower bed – tangled between a budding hawthorn and an unhealthy rose bush – winded, dizzy and shocked.

'Oh God, I'm sorry, I'm sorry,' Mark said, crouching down beside me. He looked pretty shaken but I could tell part of him wanted to laugh. 'Are you OK?'

'I'm fine,' I muttered, and let him detach the claws of the rose bush and haul me to my feet. He steadied me on the flat while I rubbed my head and inspected the mud on my jeans, the grazes on my elbows, the gravel stones embedded in my hands. I wiped my forehead with the back of my hand. It was streaked with blood from a scratch.

'You should have filmed that for *You've Been Framed*,' I said. 'You might have won fifty quid.' My voice was shaky. I didn't know whether to laugh or cry. So I did both. It was progress of sorts.

45

Progress there may have been, but I couldn't escape thoughts of suicide. The possibility that I might be able to free myself from the shame and torment that controlled me was, absurdly, my main motivation for getting up in the morning. Finding an acceptable way to kill myself, however, was proving more of a challenge than I had anticipated. Not least because I had ruled out the majority of methods. The removal of all dangerous weaponry from the house and restrictions on the quantity of prescription drugs I was permitted at any one time eliminated two of the most straightforward ways. Plus, after the fiasco with the kitchen knife and being naturally a bit of a wimp, I had rejected anything too violent or potentially painful. Likewise, I didn't want the risk of harming a bystander, or surviving but leaving myself seriously injured. Which – even if I hadn't had my driving licence confiscated by the DVLA – meant I wasn't planning on crashing the car. With my luck, I'd kill an innocent party instead of myself. I imagined myself with crush injuries and confined to a wheelchair, begging deaf ears for a second chance to end it all just to relieve the guilt. Jumping off a building or a bridge weren't top of my list either.

Water might look like a soft landing, but from fifty metres you may as well be jumping onto concrete. Two broken legs would rule out physio gym sessions for a while and I relied on the physical and mental respite they gave me. I briefly considered firearms, but getting my hands on a gun might be tricky, and with my tremor, I'd certainly misfire, maybe take off my ear or shoot the neighbour's dog. An overreactive gag reflex and an aversion to choking were more than enough to put me off hanging myself, and anyway I worried in case it would be drawn out, or I survived brain-injured, and Mark had to wipe my bum for the rest of his life. Someone had once told me that drowning wasn't too unpleasant (although how they had acquired that particular piece of information I had never thought to ask, for they had patently not carried it through themselves), but I knew that if my body wasn't found for a while, it would become bloated and mutilated and nibbled by fish, and I didn't want Mark to see me like that. Vain, even to the end. Plus I didn't want to be too hot, too cold or too sick. Basically, if Goldilocks had been suicidal, she would have been me.

46

'I'm a plodder,' John Lamb told me one day, as if it was something to be proud of. We were discussing work. How I defined myself by it. How driven I was and how fearful I was of losing that drive. How anything less than perfection was basically failure. Who I thought I had to prove myself to. And how I had been counting on the baby to make me re-evaluate it all.

But a plodder? The idea was horrific. John Lamb was top of his game. Well known and respected. Prestigious. I had him down as a high-flier. Not someone who would boast of his mediocrity.

He laughed. 'You know, sometimes, Helen, good enough is good enough.'

I practically choked. Every piece of wisdom that he had imparted, every practical technique he had taught me, all the work we had ever done, it all came crashing down around my ears. Everything he had ever told me had to be re-evaluated in light of this latest revelation. The evidence was irrefutable. The man had completely lost his mind.

I met Newly Qualified Nicola from Ferguson House at the station on my way home from one of my sessions. She trapped me before I had time to take flight. I didn't want to chat. Especially not with her.

'Oh, hi,' I said, but she refused to take my surliness in the manner it was intended. My foul mood wasn't a general one. It was specific and targeted. I hadn't forgiven her for toying with me on the ward.

She'd left nursing, she told me. Sued the hospital because one of the male patients had attacked her. Practically bitten off her ear, she claimed, and it had taken months to heal. The ward manager had been negligent in leaving her alone with him. Now she was working as a barmaid in a bar near to the station and, honestly, she couldn't believe how much she was enjoying it. She'd had it with patients, with nursing, the whole lot. Despite the dig, despite my own fairly wretched state, I pitied her. I knew, if I cared to, I'd surely discover she'd been sacked.

But, honestly, I didn't care to.

I let her lies wash over me. I plastered on a smile and moved along the platform. And took a later train home.

47

Much of the time, it wasn't the past that haunted me so much as the future that hadn't happened. I wasted hours asking myself what had become of the person I was supposed to be. Hours wondering if the child we hadn't had would have led us elsewhere. To a place where I hadn't had a breakdown. A place where I had held work and life together. Where I wasn't feeble and pathetic. But Geraldine told me there was no point in thinking like that. No point in going over and over it. No point in ruminating. That's what my thoughts were. Ruminations. I pictured a cow chewing my brain, regurgitating it, chewing it again. Regrets and shame and guilt spewing out.

48

The last two weeks of May were glorious. Geraldine left and was replaced by Evelyn. Despite my difficulties with new people, I took the change in my uncoordinated stride. Geraldine had been assigned to me on a recommendation from Lorraine, and neither of us had wanted to disappoint her. We had smiled at each other a lot, been courteous and considerate to one another because that was what nice people did, and she had given me valuable practical and psychological support. I couldn't fault her. But we were not friendly. We had not connected in any deeper way. To pre-empt my own feelings of inadequacy and because I was convinced that she would never take to me, I had secretly branded Geraldine as one of those high-maintenance women who thought their appearance was a measure of their worth. She was always perfectly turned out: clothes, hair, makeup, soft-top car. Everything I wasn't. But my judgement was unfair and untrue. She was professional in every way. We just didn't click.

Evelyn, though, was different. She was small, dark-haired, direct. Straight off, she ducked under my barriers and plonked herself next to me on the sofa rather than in the armchair across the coffee-table divide as Geraldine had done. Curled in on myself on the outside and the inside, I sat there shaking, my crossed feet nervously tapping the base of the sofa while she chatted freely about her kids and her husband and the work they were doing on their house, and gradually, as I realised she wasn't going to demand anything of me that I wouldn't be able to give, I began to unfurl. It occurred to me, not for the first time, how much a therapeutic relationship depended on the particular personalities involved. The fact that I'd had so many run-ins with staff on the ward and elsewhere didn't say much about my personality. On the other hand, it spoke volumes about Evelyn. Either she actually liked me, or she was extremely good at faking it.

But even with Evelyn by my side, I was still struggling. Not only was the path to recovery so steep that most of the time I couldn't even face putting on my hiking boots, never mind find the energy to scale it without slipping backwards, but it was also pitted with crevasses that I fell into on more than one occasion. Evelyn was quick to spot any deterioration and acted fast, either by tweaking my medication or by getting me seen by the consultant. Although I had promised Dr L that his crummy ward was the last place I'd be coming back to, I had a couple of short admissions for top-up ECT. The admissions were planned, a day or two for treatment with no hanging around afterwards. By all accounts (even mine), it seemed I was making reluctant progress. But rather than this progress being welcome, it horrified me. It reinforced just how low I had fallen, how far I still had to go, how awful the whole process was and would still be for anyone close to me. The summit didn't seem worth aiming for. The view made me vertiginous and sick. I seriously doubted that it was worth the pain of dragging myself over the scree to get there. Superficially I might have begun to function better, but the wounds inside me were still raw, and I could not even vaguely comprehend how they would ever heal.

49

For my birthday in June, Mark took me to a country hotel in the Highlands. What should have been a treat was a massive psychological and physical challenge. To date, I hadn't dared stay overnight in a strange bed. I clung to the safety of my own home and the comfort of the cat, and had to be cajoled into undertaking this adventure. It went as could have been predicted. As we pulled through the imposing gates and headed up the sweeping driveway, I was begging Mark to take me home. Outside the hotel, a parking valet – uniformed and politely stiff – allowed us to finish our discussion as if it was normal for the guests to arrive in tears, and took the keys to our ageing electric-blue Micra (we had yet to take Billy's advice and upgrade) with a deference that implied all their clientele drove such shite cars. Inside, the hotel was an intimidatingly swish mix of traditional and trendy. It could have – probably had – featured in a design magazine. The vast hallway had a huge fireplace with a roaring fire too hot for the weather and a mantelpiece where one could lean one's elbow as one smoked one's cigar or stroked one's hipster beard before such things had even existed. High ceilings with elaborate cornices and Art

Nouveau lamps watched over antique armchairs, revamped with the latest Harris-tweed upholstery in tasteful shades of heather, and coffee-table books of the latest architectural fashions. Stags' heads squinted at us from between abstract canvases as if they were in on the irony and not at all dead.

While Mark checked in, I made a beeline for the toilets. It wasn't just my mental state making everything such an ordeal. My stomach was cramping, in part from nerves but mainly due to my latest bout of constipation. Constipation as a word, however, did not do justice to the agony that I was suffering. The culprit was lithium and it had been causing me varying degrees of discomfort since way back. I regularly took lactulose or other laxatives to help, but this particular spell was threatening to require explosives. After several minutes of undignified straining, which failed yet again to provide any relief, I gave up and washed my hands. I was too jittery and in too much pain to appreciate the classy toiletries and impeccably white hand-towel squares rolled into precise cigars and perfectly aligned in a basket. I avoided the mirror and dried my hands on the back of my jeans.

The door of our room was heavy, stained oak and opened with a mortice key. Mark unlocked it with a flourish. He stood back to let me enter first. I was met by a bed of majestic proportions furnished with an excessive number of pillows, a variety of cushions serving no particular purpose other than inconvenience and enough bed throws to blanket Loch Ness. At the far end of the room was an Art Deco cocktail trolley bearing a silver tray on which there was a bottle of wine (that I later noted was not complimentary) and two glasses, and a tasteful console with a television three times the size of our new Sony at home. I perched on the edge of the bed and tugged off my trainers. I wanted to sink into the plush carpet and lose myself in the generous folds of the curtains, or hide under the feather duvet and bury my head in the billowing pillows. But I couldn't. I couldn't relax. I was twitchy and in agony, and convinced that, upstream of the blockage, my guts were being inflated by the bellows that I'd seen in the hearth in the downstairs hallway.

'Check out the en-suite,' Mark said. 'You could have a bath.' I could hear how desperate he was to make me happy. I dragged myself off the bed. The bathroom was a slate and chrome affair. Sleek, glass-panelled walk-in shower, contemporary free-standing bath. It was far removed from the rickety plastic flap on the shower-over-the-bath and black grout in our bathroom at home. We had intended to redo it as soon as we had moved in. Three years down the line, it was in as bad a state as ever. Life, or whatever it was we'd been going through, had got in the way of the refurb.

'Can I have a minute?' I begged, and closed the door behind me.

'OK?' Mark asked when I reappeared.

'Fine,' I lied.

Pre-dinner drinks were served in the conservatory. I'd put on a black dress that I'd bought in London when I was a couple of months pregnant. When I'd bought it, my pregnancy boobs had filled it. Now it sagged over my non-existent tits and even my bloated stomach couldn't disguise the jut of my pelvic bones. I tottered my way down the carpeted staircase in foolish three-inch heels, narrowly avoiding a sprained ankle. Not for the first time, I reflected on the multiple and inventive ways my body had – and continued to – let me down.

In the conservatory, I clutched my gin and tonic. Despite the light, the glass, the air, I was suffocating. I was terrified of spilling my drink, of breaking the crystal glass. Terrified of my tremors giving me away, of alcohol flushes. Terrified of all the other guests. I put the drink down. It was too much.

'I need to go outside,' I whispered to Mark. He took my hand and led the way. Outdoors, the cool air soothed me, but my body still shook and my heels sunk into the moss lining the gaps between the paving stones, so we sat on a limestone wall, holding hands, drinking in the tinge of sea salt on the air and listening to the evening song of wood pigeons and warblers. It was almost midsummer, and the evening was filled with that special Scottish light, a light near bright as daylight but somehow subdued by the scent of dusk and dew and lush greenery, and by vanilla-sweet broom and the throat-catching must of wild redcurrant, and our shadows thinned so much they could not be seen. The midges that usually thicken the Highland air were scarce and scattered, and danced for us in the last low sunrays. And at our feet, the otherwise perfectly manicured lawn muddied by molehills faded in the gloaming.

At the dining table, I sat in the straight-backed chair with rigid formality, trying to outdo the cramping in my gut, and flinched when the waiter flicked open my napkin. I picked at the fancy food and shoved it around the plate. I gulped down water and glasses of wine.

Before breakfast the next morning, after a restless night

in the king-size bed, we made an emergency trip to the pharmacy in Oban. Despite my medical training and my familiarity with the vagaries of the human body, I was always mortified asking for laxatives. *Yes, Dulcolax. Yes, suppositories. Yes, I know where they go.*

50

Further progress.

'Fifty-six pence, please.'

I handed over the money. I was in the 7-Eleven in our local shopping parade, testing the mechanics of acquisition. Testing how many paracetamol tablets I could buy in a single trip out of the house.

It was one of the few times I had walked up to the shops alone. Mark and Evelyn would have been proud of my progress, but it was a cheap deception. After the 7-Eleven I was heading to the newsagent, both pharmacies and the small supermarket. A couple of boxes from each and I'd be sorted. The ease of it gave me a rush of exhilaration. The law around the amount that could be sold in a single transaction had recently come into force and I had easily outwitted it. It was the first time in two years that I had been in control.

The truth was, though, that I wasn't going to kill myself with paracetamol. As an on-call senior house officer years before, I'd seen enough overdoses with the drug to know how unpleasant it could be. Monitoring blood levels, titrating the antidote, the patient teetering on the brink of fulminating liver failure. And when it came, a tortuous, torturous death, often with the patient conscious and with time enough to regret their decision. I didn't want the chance to have regrets. I certainly didn't want to discover that I'd changed my mind when it was too late. Imagine having a life-yearning epiphany when you were too far gone to go back. Fuck that.

By the time I got home, the pills were rattling my nerves. In a flurry of contrition, I confessed to John Lamb. He suggested that I hand my hoard over to Mark. For once, I took his advice.

After the paracetamol subterfuge, my medication was rationed to daily prescriptions. Every day except Sundays, I had to collect my meds from the local pharmacy. On Saturdays I received double the dose, but Mark was charged with guarding the extras. Derek, the pharmacist, was gentle with me even when I let my irritation show. Which was, of course, all the time. He tried his hardest to lessen my humiliation by looking out my drug pack the moment he spotted me. He let me skip the queue, always asked how I was doing without expecting an answer. When he wasn't there, it was mortifying. The other pharmacists would call back to their colleagues who were working at the dispensing hoods, counting, checking, packaging pills. 'Is today's pack ready for Dr Taylor?' It was worse if there was a locum and I had to explain. Before risking an approach, I'd hide behind shelves of home blood-pressure monitors or medicated dandruff shampoo and wait for the other customers to leave.

'Daily? That's very unusual. Are you sure?'

Of course I was sure. Fucking moron.

51

Summer began to fade. The acer tree flamed and the evening sun hung lower in the sky. September tinged the air with a subtle melancholy – the drawing-in of the summer days, a certain aspect to the sunlight, the mouldering smell of the approaching autumn and the threat of the anniversaries it heralded.

52

'I'll take them,' I said, admiring myself in the foot mirror, turning this way and that. The trainers were light-blue leather, with fine stitching and bobbly moulded soles. The mirror showed a peek of light-grey trainer sock, black-legging Lycra over my stick legs, the purple hem of my Jigsaw dress.

The shop owner rang them up and I card-swiped without flinching. Pricier than my usual but worth the money. I bit my cheek to tame the stupid grin that threatened to burst across my face. I wanted to hug myself for being so clever, so cunning. If anyone was watching me, they would be completely fooled. Buying expensive trainers was not the move of someone who was about to kill themselves.

I was practised now in the art of deceit. For most of my depression, I'd been too weak to put up a front. Hadn't had the wherewithal to fool anyone. But recently, I had stopped being so open about the way that I felt. For weeks, I'd been lying to Mark and Evelyn, to my family, to my friends, to John Lamb and Dr Hargreaves. Persuading them that I was out of the danger zone.

Outside, I practically skipped along the pavement, swinging the branded carrier bag. This was the start of something new, something big. I knew exactly what I was going to do. I had used my medical knowledge to come up with an invincible plan. It would be irresponsible to detail precisely what it was, but I had worked out how to get hold of a dangerous non-prescription drug in a dose that no one had ever survived and invented a plausible reason for requesting such an excessive quantity. I didn't want Derek implicated in my plot, though, so I popped into the other pharmacy in the shopping arcade where they didn't know me. Where, as far as they knew, I was as sane as any normal person.

In the pharmacy, I spouted my story with barely a hesitation. I might have been thin, shaky and pale, but I was grinning like a maniac and I had new trainers. When the pharmacist went through the back to the prep room, I moseyed around the shop, testing eyeliners on the back of my hand and checking out the lipsticks. I never wore lipstick. It probably wasn't the moment to start. And then he was back, shoving the box into a paper bag, and I was settling up and heading back home. Inside, I was whooping. If my singing voice had been less tortured, I would have burst into song.

At home, I plonked myself in the middle of the living-room floor, took my new trainers out of their box and admired them. I sniffed the fresh leather and ran my fingers over the bobbles on their soles. Then I placed them back in the box and slipped the box back into the carrier bag. For safety, I stapled the receipt to the bag. That way, when Mark returned them, he'd be sure to get a full refund.

Everything was more or less ready. Inside the pharmacy paper bag, screwed tightly at its neck where I had been gripping it, was a small, plain cardboard box labelled with a sticker giving the expiration date and the modest instructions on how to take the drugs, and inside the box, the blister packs of tablets rasping against each other. I was shaking as usual and it was fear, but not the draining, enervating fear that I was so used to. It was how I imagined I might feel at the top of a ski slope, an energising, exhilarating fear, the type of fear you get from speed and risk, the type of uplifting fear that thrives on danger. And it was a thirst too, made more acute by anticipation. And me, desperate for the relief of quenching it.

The cat scuppered it all. She nosed past the living-room door and chirruped when she found me sitting on the floor.

'Hello, baby,' I said, holding out my fingers for her to rub against. She approached, nuzzled, let me rub her ears. She let me pick her up, and I stood, catching our reflection in the window, her face against mine, her paws over my shoulder. And I was saturated with the smell of her, her fur, her whiskers, the squidgy bit at the side of her mouth. Her claws were digging into my shoulder, gripping and releasing in time with her purrs. Something broke inside me. I put her down and started to cry.

'Catkins,' I said. I couldn't tell her what I was planning to do. I couldn't cope with her bewilderment. My intent began to unravel.

Reluctantly, I phoned the clinic. Asked to see someone urgently. Dr Hargreaves wasn't available but one of her senior house officers was there.

In the treatment room, she questioned me, examined me and took a blood sample to check my lithium levels. I told her that I had a plan but I didn't tell her how close I was to putting it into action. She popped out of the room to phone Dr Lorimer. I sat on the edge of the bed, swinging my feet, studying the sterile packs on the treatment trolley and counting the yellow sharps bins. When she returned, she explained that they had decided that it wasn't appropriate to readmit me. It had taken me so long to get out after the first admission. I was doing so well. It would be a terrible shame to go backwards.

I hopped down from the bed.

'But I'm going to kill myself,' I said.

I guess they had heard it all before.

53

At the station waiting for the train home, I burned with mortification. I had completely humiliated myself by asking for help. Help that I hadn't even been sure I wanted. What a joke I was. What an absolute total joke. The doctor had completely got the measure of me. She'd said I could come to the clinic again the next day and she'd make an emergency appointment for me to see John Lamb, but it didn't make me feel any less stupid. And I raged against her and Dr L even while knowing they were right. On the ward, I'd become institutionalised and dependent. I was feeble and utterly pathetic. Laughable and infantile.

By the time the train arrived at my stop, I was incandescent with shame and self-loathing. I jumped off the train. For once my legs flew. I ran home. Leapt up the garden steps. Flung open the front door. The smell of bleach smacked me straight in the face. Sandra was in. Shit. I'd forgotten the day.

I mumbled a hi and scarpered upstairs, too fired up to be ashamed of my abruptness.

'Almost done,' she called after me.

Upstairs, I rummaged in my knicker drawer for the

stash of lorazepam that I had hidden from Mark. For the last few weeks, I'd been taking half doses to build up a stock. It wasn't a drug that was going to kill me, but it would take the edge off whatever else might happen. In my bedside cabinet I uncovered a few sleeping pills that had escaped his notice. Downstairs, I heard Sandra putting the vacuum cleaner back in the cupboard. Not long now. She always finished off with the bathroom on the landing. The moment I heard the whirr of the extractor fan, I tore downstairs, grabbed the other drugs, a bottle of gin and a bowl, and rushed into the back garden. I didn't say goodbye to the cat.

Outside, I scrambled up the slope until I reached the garden bench. There, hidden by rhododendron bushes and a tangle of brambles, I punched out my stash into the bowl. I let the pills run between my fingers like sand. Untwisted the lid of the gin and sniffed. The fumes mingled with the cloying scent of wild garlic that grew in abundance under the oaks in the copse behind.

I took a lip-pursed sip and waited for Sandra to leave.

I didn't have to wait long. A few minutes later I heard her cheery call to me. I didn't answer. I felt churlish and rude and guilty. Then, at long last, I heard the swing of the gate and I was alone.

Immediately, I took a huge swig of gin and grabbed a handful of pills. Shoved them in my mouth. Dry-gulped them down. My stomach leapt past my heart. A fleeting thought that I should have brought water, but after two years of practice I was an expert at taking tablets. I could swallow handfuls with just a mouthful of liquid. I took another gin swig, another handful, another and another. A state of calm crept over me, enveloped me, and I leaned back on the bench and stared at the sky. Listened to the peace. And to the stillness of the garden disturbed only by the crawl of snails across grass stems, the scratch of ant feet on the path, the suckling of bees in the snapdragons.

This is what I think happened next.

I finished the pills. Then I phoned Mark to tell him that I loved him.

Woozy, calm, I must have staggered back down the garden – past the acer tree blazing in the late-summer sunshine – rolled up at the back door and gone inside to get the phone.

'No, Helen. No.' He knew. Straight away he knew. He had been dreading this day for two years or more.

'It's OK,' I said. 'It'll all be OK.'

I remember standing under the whirligig washing line. The peg bag was hanging from it but there was no washing to bring in. I remember sitting at the bottom of the steps where I had taken a tumble a few months before, looking at the daisies scattered on the patch of lawn. Stars in a galaxy. I remember digging a hole in the path with a twig.

And next thing, one of our best friends was there. An ambulance arrived. Mark too. The paramedics escorted me out of the garden. Past the waxy rhododendrons gleaming in the late afternoon. Over the pink gravel chips that jammed into the rubber soles of my Converse. And me, stumbling. Giggling foolishly. As if I had been caught smoking behind the bike sheds.

Our friend came with me in the ambulance. I remember clambering in the back, pleased that I wouldn't die at home and taint the house for Mark. I had succeeded. This was all a formality. Mark followed in the car. Trailing the ambulance. Panicked and sick. The traffic at a crawl. The paramedics didn't blue-light me. They didn't induce vomiting or pump my stomach. I was pissed. I was laughing. They assumed I was a time-waster.

At the Western, I was taken into resus. Our friend was with me, holding my hand, willing me on. Mark wasn't there yet. He was parking the car. Driving in circles, stricken, blind with terror. The house officer tried to put a line in. The veins on the back of my hand were set solid, twists of cable wire, blocked from the number of anaesthetics I'd had for ECT. I told them. Giggling. Teasing them. Taking the piss. You won't manage. It's OK. I was drifting. It doesn't matter. Honestly. It's fine. Drifting. Smiling. Fading.

Gone.

54

They didn't think I would last the night. Mark was told to prepare himself. That's all I know.

In the black hole of a coma, there is no measure of time. Eventually, I saw a halo. It was my sister's blonde hair, backlit by a rare perfusion of sunshine and diffracted by the striae of my flickering eyelashes. She may have looked like an angel, but something about the scratch of my hospital gown and the sensation of gagging on the ventilator tube suggested I wasn't actually in heaven.

'Hello,' she said. Tenderly. As if I was a child she had woken from sleep.

Mark held my hand as the nurses took out the tube.

I wanted to cry. I hadn't been afraid of death. I figured that it couldn't be any more taxing than before I was born. But I was afraid of this.

'I'm sorry,' I whispered. 'I'm sorry.' The steady beep of monitors and the rasp of ventilators betrayed the dissonance of my words. For I was sorry, but not in the way I should have been. I was sorry I was still there, sorry for failing, sorry for the disruption I had caused. Sorry that I wasn't sorry for what I had done. I made my apologies again and again. Mark gazed at the opposite wall. My sister nodded. It was true that I was sorry for the pain I had put them through, which I could read on their drawn faces and in the words that wouldn't come. But it was an intellectual regret, a regret manifest in thoughts rather than emotions. I was too distraught to have the capacity to feel their pain.

I'm sorry. They were words repeated to Geraldine and Evelyn when they came to see me, to Dr Lorimer, to Dr Hargreaves, to John Lamb. To the rest of my family and my friends. Words that were necessary to hide the truth. Words that prompted John Lamb to conclude that I was relieved I hadn't succeeded, was glad that I had survived, that what I had been aiming for was not death but an escape from the person that I had been. But he was wrong. I wasn't relieved. And how could I ever escape myself?

For the next few days I drifted in and out of consciousness. Gradually, the nip of the cannulae, the catch of the central line in my neck, the drag of the urinary catheter tugged me back. Item by item, the equipment was turned off, the drips and infusions removed. I even requested the urinary catheter be taken out. But then I needed to pee.

'There isn't a toilet,' the nurse told me. 'Our patients aren't usually well enough.' Even in ICU, I was a fraud. A bedpan was retrieved from the next ward but it wasn't up to the job. I was several litres overhydrated and my aim wasn't great. The warmth creeping up my back and a spreading damp patch on the sheets were a giveaway of my misfire. Mortification almost succeeded in finishing me off where the overdose had failed. The nurse stripped the wet sheets and helped me change my hospital gown. And yet again, I felt like an infant.

A little later, the consultant came to see me. He told me how near I had come to dying, how I had the highest-ever recorded level of the toxin in my system, how I should not have survived.

'Really?' I said, sensing an opportunity. 'In that case, I might write myself up.' I meant in an academic article for a medical or scientific publication. As I explained, I was always on the lookout for another research paper or two.

He regarded me with horror. It was clearly not a subject to joke about.

Mark reads this chapter and tells me that isn't what happened. His voice wavers. 'You didn't say sorry.'

'What? What did I say?'

'You said *oh no*.'

I knew that had been my first thought when I'd woken but I had convinced myself I wouldn't have been so cruel as to say the words out loud. I say sorry and mean it this time. I cry. He cries too.

55

A friend asked me why I did it. When there were people who loved me. When there were people I loved. Whether I thought it was selfish and whether I felt any guilt. Those weren't her words, but the meaning was clear. What she actually said was, 'Did you still feel like you?'

I think she wanted me to say no. To say that I had been taken over by a stranger and that I didn't know who I was. That way, I wouldn't have to bear the responsibility and she wouldn't have to judge me for what I had done. But it wasn't the case. However lost I had been, inside I was always me.

56

From ICU, I went straight to Ferguson House. Despite physical complications resulting from the strain on my heart and kidneys, none of the medical wards were willing to take me. I was a psychiatric patient and the psychiatrists were getting me back. There, I was put in a six-bedded room. Mine was one of the two beds nearest the corridor, so the staff could keep an eye on me from outside the room. It was the worst place to be. Neither daylight nor privacy. Between me and the natural light, a barrier of curtained beds hid their occupants. And when I pulled my curtains round to hide, Gentle John or Amanda would spring to their feet and swish them open.

I was too broken to protest. Physically and mentally, I was a mess. Fluid had settled in my lungs and was hindering my breathing. My legs were swollen up to my thighs with oedema. I had scabs on my neck and in my groin from the cannulae. All my medication had been stopped because of the risk to my heart. I couldn't shift the congestion in my lungs despite physiotherapy and nebulisers. When I lay down, a cough racked my body and aggravated my bruised sternum. When I stood up too quickly, I passed out. I had no diazepam to dampen my anguish. No antidepressants to soften my despair. No antipsychotics to relieve my paranoia or my sense of persecution.

Although I was on constant, my keepers were slightly less vigilant than they had been on my first admission, perhaps because I was so physically unwell. I took whatever escape I could. When they weren't paying attention, I'd crawl into the toilets and lock the door. It was a risky strategy. Plumbing problems were a constant. Ferguson House and its fellows were never meant to be permanent and their systems had not been built to cope. Pipes that had too narrow a gauge, with too shallow a slope, and too much demand. The loo in my single room had just about coped. In the six-bedders, they were constantly blocked. Odd socks, plastic bags, drug beakers. And shit. More than once, the stench had me vomiting over the filthy pan. But even when they were clean, I never had the chance to hang around for long. Someone would be after me, hammering on the door, threatening to open it from the outside and drag me back to my bed.

Across the room from me was a well-to-do, sixty-something lady called Marjory. Each morning she rose at 7.30 a.m. prompt and put her silky gown over her nightdress. Then, with her sponge bag tucked under her arm, she braved the showers and chanced the roulette that was the toilets. When she was done, she would blow-dry, tong and pin up her hair, dress in a tweed skirt and blouse with a fitted jacket, and do her careful makeup. From the overheard conversations with the other patients and the nurses, I gathered she had been admitted with depression after the death of her husband but, from the way she spoke, I reckoned she was mourning the loss of her looks more than the loss of her spouse. This was her first time in Ferguson

House – previously she'd been in the Priory and the standards here were not what she was used to – and it was clear she was having difficulty adapting. And not just to Ferguson House. It seemed her husband had done everything for her. Except, perhaps, tonging her hair.

I condemned her with my silent judgement. Someone with all the advantages in life and none of the wherewithal to put them to good use.

One night she heard me sobbing in the dark.

'Are you all right, dear?' She came over and stood by my bed. 'I know you don't like to talk to us, but I'm here if you need me.'

My soul withered in shame.

57

Summer holidays as a kid were a fortnight in August on the Isle of Arran in a tumbledown cottage with a bath hidden under a wooden trapdoor in the kitchen and a spider-infested outside toilet. They were holidays of Irn-Bru-and-wasp picnics, terry-towelling shorts and matching hoodies, somersaults on the beach trampolines, and a perilous hike up Goat Fell in flip-flops. And sometimes Dad would hire a rowing boat and the four of us kids would take it in turns to go out with him in pairs with our hand-lines to fish for mackerel. While Dad rowed, we'd hang over the end of the boat with the oars splashing beside us and feel the drag of the lines across the water and let ourselves be hypnotised by the dip and swell of the sea. If you stared hard enough, you could just make out the twinkle of the tin-foil lures attached to the hooks nearest the surface. I was always astonished at how quickly the depths darkened. And then, suddenly, there'd be a tug of the line and we'd wake from our trance and wind in the hand-lines, and there they'd be, twisting flashes of green-silver, muscle tails thrashing, pierced mouths gagging. Unhooked, they would slip between our fingers as we tried to grab them before they leapt back into the waves. But before long, their iridescence dulled and they flipped and flopped around the bottom of the boat, puncture wounds oozing, eyes drying, gills flaring.

The events of the previous week had left me as desperate and floundering as those dying fish. I was counting on Lorraine to sort me out. Although what that meant, what I thought she might be able to do for me, whether it meant flinging me back in the sea or putting me out of my misery, I could not have properly explained.

When she came back after her days off, it did not go as expected. Not at all. I had hoped we might pick up where we'd left off, with anecdotes and sick jokes and a gentle teasing for my failed attempt after my insistent bragging that any plan I'd come up with would be foolproof. Anything to take my mind off my miserable state. But when I approached her, she brushed me off with a smile. It left me reeling. I couldn't understand why she no longer had the time for me. I analysed every interaction we had ever had, ruminated on why I'd been snubbed, wondered what on earth I had done. Much later (and once the damage had been done), I discovered that she had been instructed by her superiors not to consort with me. After my first long stay, they considered that we had become too close. That I had become too dependent.

Without Lorraine, I was forced to look elsewhere.

I had met Kieran, another staff nurse, a week or so before I'd been discharged the first time and on the few occasions that I'd been readmitted for extra ECT sessions. He was cool, sensible, well trained and thoroughly decent. He'd always been kind whenever I'd needed him before. I tracked him down to a side room. I stood in the doorway like a lemon.

'Hi, Kieran.'

He glanced up from the dressing trolley he was preparing. 'Yes,' he said. 'What is it?' Unsaid but clearly heard: *Can't you see I'm busy?*

My blood flashed glacial in my veins. Icy fingers twanged the tendons in the back of my neck. I knew the feeling. Fear, stress, foolishness, whatever it is that happens when you know you've upset someone. Especially if it is someone you like and respect. But desperation overpowered the grip of fear so I kept on.

'Do you have a moment to talk at all?' I was begging. I could hear it in the shallow gasps between my words.

'Sorry, Helen. I'm busy.' *For fuck's sake. Are you blind or what?*

'Later maybe?'

He sighed and looked up. 'Another time? It's pretty hectic today.' All I could hear was contempt, judgement, disgust. *I don't have time for fakers and attention-seekers.*

As a child, I would turn away from the suffocating panic of the dying fish, but I still felt the thuds when Dad struck their heads against the prow of the rowing boat. Bashing their brains out on the wood until our catch was reduced to a pool of blood and the dead twitch of tails and gills.

Kieran hadn't laid a finger on me, but he may as well have bashed my brains out. I limped back to my room, dragging my shame with me.

Dr L chucked me out the moment I could stand without passing out. Back home I paced from room to room and waited for Mark to return from work. I'd slept off my diazepam dependence while I'd been in a coma but it was proving difficult to get through each day without something to take the edge off.

As flukes go, that I had survived at all was pretty major. That I had survived without any clinically significant consequences was totally off the scale. Once it was clear my heart hadn't been damaged, my antidepressants were gradually reintroduced. But I can't say I noticed much difference.

58

In many ways, the weeks and months that followed were a repeat of the months after my initial discharge. Depression, anxiety, paranoia, self-loathing. The difference was that this time I was utterly defeated. Without my plan, I had no direction. Without my plan, I lost the certainty that I would eventually win.

I went on living because I didn't have an alternative. I didn't have an epiphany. I didn't reach a state of transcendence. I didn't decide life was suddenly worth living or realise how close I had come to wasting it. It was a reflex as unthinking as breathing that dragged me through each day.

It was the very worst of times. It was hard to face what I had done to Mark and to my family and to my friends. I couldn't fathom why they didn't hate me as much as I hated myself. How they could even tolerate being near me after how badly I had let them down. Especially as I had treated the whole thing as a bad joke. But even amid my raging paranoia, I could detect only love. It seemed that life had its hooks into me and it wasn't about to let me go. I went on living because I didn't have the fight left to do otherwise.

*

Not long after discharge, my sister came for one of her regular visits with her girls. They were playing outside while we talked. I'd written goodbye notes of love to them in a notebook but they hadn't been read. For this, I was glad. I wasn't sure whether they had fully understood what had happened. Whether they might think what I had done was a betrayal. Whether they could forgive me. We didn't talk about it. Maybe they didn't even know. They are adults now. I've never dared ask them.

'Can I ask something of you, Helen?' my sister said over a cup of tea.

I nodded. I'd have done anything for her. Anything that I could.

'We're going on holiday next week. I don't want to have to worry about you.' She was on the brink of tears. 'Can you promise me that I won't have to worry about you?'

I promised. Of course I promised. But I hadn't understood the question. What I was promising was that it was OK for her not to be there all the time, it was OK for her to have some headspace without my traumas, it was OK for her not to spend every waking hour worrying about me. It was a recognition of how much she had done for me, how much of a toll it had taken. It was my attempt not to be a burden. What I was promising her was that she could go away and relax and enjoy herself and I wouldn't mind. I wouldn't mind if her thoughts strayed away from me. I wouldn't mind if it was all too much. She shouldn't need my permission to have the right not to worry. I wanted her to be free of me. It didn't even occur to me what she was really asking. It didn't occur that she was asking me to promise not to kill myself. I'm glad it didn't. Because that way, I didn't have to lie.

59

'I keep thinking I'll have a reaction,' I said at my next psychology appointment. 'Like delayed shock.'

John Lamb nodded. We were in a small room on the ground floor of his usual building. This one was cramped. Dark. Divided off from a larger one. Separated from the admin office and the photocopier by plasterboard walls.

'Is this your office now?'

He nodded again.

I wondered if he was miffed about the downgrade. This one had none of the grandeur of the upstairs room. None of the old furniture. Not even his comfortable armchair. He hadn't managed to shut his eyes once during this session.

'You know, a panic attack or something,' I said. 'When it sinks in properly.'

'It might come later,' he said. 'Or it might never come. It might be a protection mechanism.'

We sat in silence for a while. I surveyed the room. Appraised the spartan furniture. Thought about the other office upstairs.

'Why did you move?'

He took his usual minute before he replied. When he did, he spoke carefully. 'I'm winding down to retirement.'

'What?' I gulped. If anything was going to make me have a panic attack, it was going to be that. I had no idea how I would cope without him.

'It's OK,' he said. 'I'll keep seeing the patients I already have. I'm just not taking on anyone new.'

So that was it. The beginning of the end.

'You know, Helen,' he said after several minutes of silence. 'Some things are too momentous for our brains to comprehend.'

He wasn't wrong there.

60

Together Evelyn and Mark ganged up on me, scheming plans to bring me back to life. It took them months and months of dedicated effort. I felt weak and sick and pathetic. But I didn't have the fight left to resist. It was hard going. Slow going. I had an astronomical distance to cover and I was going at a shuffle.

Mark bought me a piano. When I couldn't do anything else, I sat at it and picked out stilted melodies until I had done it often enough to play the tunes I had learned for the exams I'd failed as a teenager.

'You're good,' Mark would say as he prepared our evening meal. It was obvious he was no musician.

Sessions with John Lamb continued in much the same way as they had before. It often felt like all I was searching for was justification for why I hadn't coped. I wanted excuses for failing at everything I had ever done. He helped me reach a better understanding of myself and, at least intellectually, reframe my failure as something less inadequate. But it didn't rid me of the terror that underneath it all I was simply faulty.

*

Without my lithium tremor, physical activity became easier. Mark and I started playing badminton with friends. I dared a drop-in netball session and didn't self-combust. I began running to get my fitness back. It wasn't quick – my pace or my recovery. Every step was painful and made me want to vomit.

A year passed. Single-handedly I was preventing John Lamb from enjoying his retirement.

For two years the future had been something that hadn't existed for me beyond the next day. Now that I had screwed up my best way out, it became something that would be hard to avoid. With no real alternative, the possibility of work formed as a vague apparition on the horizon. I went back to my books. Back to the basics of molecular biology, the essentials of malariology, the foundations of protein chemistry – knowledge that was bobbing about, lost in my macerated mind.

I was getting fitter, stronger. I started playing netball with a club. I stopped going to the physio and went back to the off-campus university gym near my house. With muscles in my arms and legs, I lost my skeletal thinness. There was little externally to set me apart. Little to identify me as anything other than perfectly normal.

A couple of friends from down south came to visit. We walked Conic Hill and the banks of Loch Lomond and drank too many cocktails at a bar in town. The next day, one of them tuned the piano by ear and played Chopin's Scherzo number 1 in B minor or something of equal drama and complexity.

'Good,' Mark said. 'But not as good as Helen.'

61

My sister came to stay for the weekend with her two girls. On Saturday night we got dressed up and went out for a meal. In the restaurant, I sat at the kids' end of the table and played 'Would you rather . . . ?' with the girls.

'Would you rather sing or fart in public?'

'Would you rather swim across a river full of crocodiles or a river full of piranhas?'

'Would you rather eat a bowl of sick or a bowl of snot?'

The three of us were helpless with laughter. Mark rolled his eyes at the bodily fluids. 'You'll get us chucked out.'

I had forgotten what it was like to laugh like that. To laugh with no control. To let go completely, without caring, and to share the moment with two little beings who I loved with every cell of my body.

When we woke on Sunday morning, the house was muffled. A foot of snow had fallen overnight. Mark and my sister went to investigate her car.

'We could dig it out but the road is blocked further up.'

If it was too hazardous to get out of our street, it was definitely too dangerous for them to attempt the two-and-a-half-hour journey back home. There was a mild panic about the girls missing their dance exams, but it was forgotten when heavy-duty bin bags came out for sledging down the embankment to the playing field. My sister and I lasted an hour max. Mark and the girls played out there until it went dark.

The next morning a slight thaw had made our road just about passable, with a helping hand. We pushed the car through the packed snow to the junction with the main road, which had been gritted, and waved them on their way.

'Do you think we should try again?' I asked as we walked back to the house.

'Sledging?' Mark said. 'Yes!'

'Not sledging, you idiot,' I said. 'IVF.' He didn't reply. I could hear the crunch of snow under his boots. I took his hand, picked at its woolly glove. 'Because, you know, I was thinking . . . the longer we wait . . .' There were puddles of meltwater under the railway bridge. The embankment to the playing field was scarred with muddy sledge runs. The snow that had been brushed from my sister's car was piled high in front of our garage. We creaked through our gate and he still hadn't said anything. Maybe he was weighing it all up. 'If we are going to do it,' I said, climbing the steps, 'maybe we should go back to the clinic in London again.' They still had the best results in the country by far. I kept talking as I unlocked the front door. If London was what we decided, I said, I was sure we could work out a way of managing the logistics. But if he was worried about money . . .

'It isn't the money,' Mark said, sitting on the stairs and pulling off his boots. 'We would find the money somehow. If we had to, we could always remortgage the house.'

'So, what do you think?' I draped my parka over the bannister. I couldn't look at him.

He stood up. 'Is that what you really want?'

'I don't know,' I said, and burst into tears. I had had such a wonderful time with my nieces. I loved them so much and longed for my own little versions, but there was so much at stake. What if we tried again and it didn't work? Or we lost another baby? But even admitting my uncertainty felt like a betrayal. Of Mark. Of the baby we lost. Of our dreams for the future. And yet, even after everything we had been through, I still wasn't quite prepared to throw away that dream for ever. I knew that if I pushed him, Mark would agree to whatever I wanted. But it probably wasn't something he would choose.

'I almost lost you.' He put his arms around me. Pulled me into him. I could hear the crack in his voice. 'I don't want to experience anything like that ever again.'

And yet . . . My sister and I had watched him and the girls for ages from the living-room window that afternoon, the three of them laughing and playing the fool. He was made to be a dad. I wanted a child for him as much as for me. I didn't know how to decide. It felt as if the right answer was out there waiting for me to choose it, but I couldn't work out what it was. Did I owe it to Mark to keep myself safe or did I owe it to him to be more resilient? Was his fear for me a good excuse for my own weakness? If I really wanted a child, shouldn't I have been strong enough to withstand whatever that meant I had to endure? I had heard of couples who had tried five, six, seven times without success. And those who had persevered and who had ultimately triumphed. I didn't know which we would be and if I could cope in either circumstance.

Later, when I talked to my sister about it, she offered to be a surrogate. I wept tears of gratitude but it wasn't the answer either. Biologically, my eggs didn't fertilise well. Although that was a major problem, it wasn't the biggest issue. I was too scared to face up to the knowledge that someone would want to do such a huge thing for me. I couldn't come to terms with how much I already owed her and I was terrified that my guilt and indebtedness would change our relationship. And, even if any of it worked, I couldn't begin to consider the burden that our longed-for child would be forced to bear simply by accident of birth. Could I lumber a child with the responsibility of giving me a reason to live, of taking the threat out of my future?

In the end, I couldn't bear the thought of hope and the lurching disappointment that would surely follow. It made me feel physically sick. We agreed. The risk was too great.

62

Months passed. I kept running. Kept playing netball. We considered adoption.

We tortured ourselves with unanswerable questions. Would we bond with the child? Would we be good parents? What if the kid had challenging behaviour? What if they didn't like us? Or we didn't like them?

We read up and tortured ourselves some more. There were rarely babies available for adoption. Most children were older than two. The academic literature told me that the first two years of a child's life were the most important for their psychological health, for that crucial bond between the mother and child. Most children came from troubled backgrounds. Drugs, alcohol, crime, abuse, incest. Except in rare circumstances, the birth family remained involved. The authorities were always searching for adoptive parents willing to take children over nine, or disabled children, or children with learning difficulties.

We discussed it and discussed it. And discussed it some more. We gave ourselves examples where adoption had been a success, and those cases where a troubled child had turned a family's life upside down. I read horror stories where couples had been forced to hand an adopted child back. Not one for looking on the bright side, I catastrophised. What would happen if it all went wrong? What if the child didn't settle with us? What if we didn't get on with the birth parents? What if their involvement was a constant reminder that we were caring for somebody else's child? What if I didn't have the capacity to love a child that wasn't mine, that wasn't Mark's? How would we cope with an older child without having had time to adjust? And what about disabilities? Or behavioural problems?

In the end, despite my inclination towards defeatism, I decided that if I could love my nieces and nephews unreservedly, and certainly if I could love the cat like a substitute offspring (although the cat wasn't a substitute anything), then perhaps it wouldn't be impossible to love someone else's child.

I made enquiries. I spoke to Janice from the council on the phone. She asked about our family situation, where we lived, what we did, whether we had any children of our own, and whether we were planning to do IVF again. I asked about age limits.

'The youngest partner should be no more than thirty-eight at the time of application.'

I was already thirty-eight. Mark was a few months older than me.

'I see.'

She asked if that was a problem. In so much as it only gave us months to get the application together and, as I told her, I hadn't been well. I explained that I was currently off work. She asked if I wouldn't mind telling her what for, that I wasn't obliged to, but it would be helpful to know. I felt the premonition of disaster. I gave an abbreviated version of the previous two years, including – mainly – the part about being sectioned and currently being under a community treatment order.

There was a telling silence.

I didn't need to listen to hear what she was about to say. With the politeness I had come to dread – the politeness of bad news – she extricated herself, thanking us for our interest and telling me that sadly I couldn't go ahead with the application when I was still under a CTO. And that even if it was lifted within the time limit, it was highly unlikely our application would succeed.

She paused, waiting for my anger.

Fake-smiling to force the words out, I said that I understood, that it wasn't her fault, and thanked her for her help.

We had been rejected before the process had even started. But the decision was correct. How could I expect to look after a vulnerable child when I could barely look after myself?

63

I made it back to work.

It took months of gentle chivvying and handholding by Mark and Evelyn, but I was back within a year of the overdose. I went through hell to get there. The alternative would have been worse though. A type of limbo where I never fully recovered yet wasn't ill enough to be numb to it. In preparation, I read scores of research papers on the latest studies on malaria parasites and their invasion of red blood cells, and took reams of notes to record the facts that wouldn't lodge in the substance of my curdled brain. Finally, I cobbled together a replacement for the project I had unwittingly abandoned more than two years earlier. I thought it amateur and unremarkable, but my boss was enthusiastic and praised my scientific thinking and my supposed capabilities, showing a belief in me that I couldn't help feeling had not been earned.

A few weeks before I was due to start back, I did a test run to the laboratory. As luck would have it, the research unit was in the process of moving into a swanky new building at the bottom of University Avenue, with sheet-glass windows and fancy lighting in the stairwell that swirled bright with neon when night fell. Unlike the old place, the new building was not haunted by ghosts of the previous me or by my memories of crying between experiments in the grim office that overlooked the bins or hiding out in the toilets when other people asked me how I was doing. Which meant, that first time, I was at least able to get myself through the front entrance.

The revolving doors spun me into the foyer. The chalky smell of dried concrete competed with vinyl glue and fresh paint. Plaster fingerprints decorated the chrome rails and doorplates. And behind closed doors, in hidden corridors, beyond the swipe-card security system that barred my way, the squeal of burning drill holes and the clang of hammers proclaimed the last of the snagging was almost complete. Fumes and dust spiralled into my lungs, and my airways clamped tight. Coughing, I fumbled in my bag for my inhaler. Once recovered, I waited at the front desk, fingering my useless security fob from the old place while shafts of sunlight sliced my eyes and a doorman I didn't recognise spoke on the phone. When he was done, he asked me to sign the visitors' book.

My boss came down to collect me. We went up two floors in the shiny lift. My reflection in the mirrored walls refused to catch my eye.

He led me to the first of two floors that our department was spread over and showed me where I'd be based – the vast empty lab, my virgin bench, the pristine culture rooms. Then he took me to the office that I was to share with a lecturer from a different department. My desk would be the one crammed into the corner. He asked me whether I thought I could work there.

'Oh, yes,' I lied. 'Totally.'

On the next floor up, the lab was busier. Several research

groups were already comfortably installed and sharing the bustling space. Centrifuges were spinning, PCR machines clicking, incubators shaking. It was a familiar soundtrack that signified countless hours dedicated to the isolation, replication and purification of the genes and proteins of the tropical parasites we were all working on. I stood for a moment in the shadows, watching the staff and students at work, listening to the easy banter and remembering the thrill of practical experiments with something akin to nostalgia. I was met with the odd half-smile and a couple of people said hi, but nobody made a great fuss or quizzed me. As far as I was concerned, I was lugging around my history on a massive sign, clear for everyone to read and judge, conspicuous in my illness, and I felt weak and invalid under the burden of it. But even had they offered, no one would have been able to take the weight from me. Most people looked past and pretended not to notice. And for that I was immensely grateful.

To ease myself in, I started back part time. I was back climbing Goat Fell in flip-flops, ill-equipped and fearful. Each morning, Mark and I drove into the West End together and he sat with me in the Italian café directly opposite my building while, sick with anxiety, I sipped an americano and made him late for work as I clung to his company for a few more desperate minutes. And when he had to go, I was four years old again, about to go to infant school.

It became clear to me very quickly that there was more to my memory loss than missing the plot of a few novels I was certain I had read or forgetting the storyline of films I wasn't completely sure that I had even seen.

I'd pass people in the corridor whose faces were acutely familiar and wonder whether to expect the greeting of a long-lost friend or the arm's-length civility of a lesser-known colleague. I learned to deal with polite enquiries without revealing my confusion.

'Helen, great to see you,' someone would say. 'How are things?'

'Yeah, really good,' I'd say. 'And you?'

Outside of work, I perfected the art of the non-introduction.

'Have you met my husband?' I'd ask when I wasn't sure who it was I was talking to and leave them to present themselves. For the most part I got away with it. But there was always the danger I might introduce someone to their own brother.

Forgetting stuff wasn't the only disorientating aspect of the damage to my memory. Time had begun to do weird things in my world. It folded back on itself and became snarled up and frayed, so I had no inherent sense of its passing. An event from a few days prior could have a distance as indistinguishable as one that had happened a year before. In the tangle, unrelated events rubbed up against each other in unexpected ways or lost the connection that they should have had.

Thankfully, my lab skills had not been ravaged in the same way. I lost myself in my experiments and hoped the rest of it would come back to me.

I made lists. I got myself a brand-new lab book, thick-tipped and fine-tipped marker pens, multicoloured rolls of labelling tape and stickers. I autoclaved pipette tips and microfuge tubes. I prepared my standard solutions, lined up the bottles on the shelf above my bench, prepared aliquots of buffers and enzymes for use in my experiments. When I had done all the procrastinating I could, I began the simplest of techniques, soothing myself with the repetition of pipetting microquantities of reagents for PCRs, running gels for the satisfaction of seeing well-defined bands of DNA, simple blots for the pleasure of discovering discrete bands on the X-ray film. Gradually, I progressed to more complicated experiments with unfamiliar equipment and protocols I hadn't tried before.

And at the end of each week, I wrote my work plans in my diary in elaborate detail so that when I came back after the weekend, I wouldn't be completely flailing.

Some mornings I couldn't do it. I couldn't control the anxiety that had me vomiting the moment I got out of bed. I couldn't summon the will to make it through the front entrance. I couldn't find the energy to carry on hiding the cracks.

The drop-in centre at ICT was still available to me. On the occasions when I phoned up in despair, Dr Hargreaves would see me if she was available. I had managed to convince myself, though, that she was irritated by my neediness, and angry because the centre had been investigated after my suicide attempt to see if they had missed any treatment opportunities. As it happens, they were cleared, but it hadn't made things any more comfortable between us. In my eyes, at least. But there was no one else I could speak to in an emergency.

I strove to convey how desperate I was.

'I'm really struggling this morning,' I'd say.

She'd listen, half-listen, send me on my way. There was not much she could do for me.

And I'd take my anxiety, my desperation, my despair back to work.

One morning, however, she came out with a self-help classic.

'You know, Helen,' she said. 'Sometimes you have to *feel the fear and do it anyway.*'

I nearly punched her fucking lights out.

64

Time progressed. Another year went by. Change was slow, but it did happen. I no longer went to ICT but saw Dr Lorimer in his clinic from time to time. He was impressed at how well I was doing. My appointments with John Lamb continued but were dwindling. Netball and work were the two main pursuits in my life. At work, I'd upped my hours to four days a week. Experiments were going well, and I was collaborating on a project with friends and former colleagues in London. I'd even managed a trip down there alone. A conference in Australia where I was planning to present the results was on the horizon and, afterwards, Mark and I were going to take a holiday there. On the netball court, I was confident, keen, fit, competitive. Fearless, even. Definitely a team player. Off court, though, I hovered at the edges and dodged potential friendships and good-natured enquiries into my life, but I think the other women just assumed I was aloof. At the age of forty, I was selected for the Scottish National Development Squad, the feeder team for the national team. It was ludicrous. From the outside, I was winning.

Inside, it was a different story. Every day was a battle. I battled to hide my memory problems. I battled to keep up appearances. And I battled ridiculous, trivial, daily anxieties that made me rage against myself.

The seminar room at the end of the corridor looked out on to the back of the hospital where I had been in intensive care, where I'd been yanked back from death, and whenever I gave a department talk or attended a lab meeting with my colleagues, it was there, staring back at me, tormenting me, challenging me, reminding me how it had almost taken me but chosen to let me go. I had been over to the other side and yet was incapable of putting things into perspective.

At home, a broken roof tile or an overdue bill was enough to trigger a crisis. A missed birthday would niggle and wake my insomnia. An appointment at the bank or a letter from human resources asking for a meeting would have me hyperventilating in anticipatory panic. If there were phone calls to be made – a car service to be arranged, a plumber to call – I made Mark do it. When it came to asking someone to do something for us, anything, paid or unpaid, professional or family, I was blocked.

At work Mark wasn't there to sort out my crap and I felt it. Anything directly related to my experiments I could just about handle. But if I had to phone for a missing order, ask the electrician to service a machine, fill out my appraisal form, or contact someone from another department to use specialised equipment, it was a nightmare. My anxiety levels were toxic. My stress in freefall.

Stressing so badly over trivialities didn't make sense. However much I tried to put the past behind me, there were daily reminders that conspired to keep it foremost in my mind – the view of the ICU in the lab meetings, bumping into patients on leave from the ward or ex-patients or nurses when I went up the street at lunchtime, passing Ferguson House on the train on my way home – but rather than forcing me to wake up to myself, all the reminders did was reinforce how pathetic my worries were now. I kept waiting for the true impact of my almost-suicide to strike because I couldn't think how else I could gain a sense of proportion. And I wanted that impact. I wanted the shock of it. Without it, I was disgusted at myself. I even found myself wishing for some terrible, external catastrophe to shock me into giving such inanities the disregard they were due. It was stupid thinking. A catastrophe would not jolt me out of my pathetic state the way the shock of ECT had jolted me from my catatonia. And the impact of such events was never fleeting. The pain always endured.

65

All my life I had dreamed of being an international athlete. For Christmas when I was nine, I was given a royal-blue tracksuit with white side-stripes and a tiny Union Jack logo on the jacket that had come from the Littlewoods Catalogue. I wore it every weekend, representing GB in gymnastics as I backflipped on an old mattress and did handsprings off the back of an old sofa, or when I captained the national netball team, whacking a ball against the outside wall of the house, sometimes recruiting my brother or younger sister as teammates or opposition, and dreaming, dreaming of having a real netball post to shoot into (instead of scoring goals by lobbing the ball onto the roof with the inherent risk of losing it up there, not to mention the possibility of breaking a roof slate and the drama that would ensue).

The first tour of the Development Squad was only a few weeks away. The final ten players who would be travelling to Dublin had yet to be announced. At a training session, we were handed leaflets with all the official advice, including information on banned substances and permitted drugs, and what to do if you were on prescription medication. I don't know whether it was that – because it would mean having to admit to the manager and coaches what I'd been going through – or whether it was the thought of having to go away from home with people I didn't know very well, or whether it was that old fear of not making the grade, of not being selected, but I wimped out. I stopped going to the training sessions. I still went to the club ones but came up with excuses not to make the others. It was the basic lesson for every could-have-been contender: you can't fail if you don't try.

At work, though, I had conned my boss into believing I still had it. But everything about me was a charade. The impression I gave was of someone tranquil, serene and quietly spoken. Hard-working, earnest, self-assured. Fuck knows how I pulled it off. It was about as far removed from the truth as Ferguson House was from a five-star hotel. Only Mark saw the wailing fits, the vertiginous attacks of PMT, the savagery of my depression. And the hideous, spiralling, nauseating insecurity.

Gradually, I slipped back into my old thought patterns. At work, once or twice a day, I unlocked the cupboard under the fume hood to check the supply of toxic chemicals. I'd move the bottles around simply to touch them, to make the connection, to reassure myself that they were there should the need arise. Ready for the day when I couldn't hold it together any more.

Madeleine McCann went missing. A three-year-old snatched from a holiday apartment in Portugal and never seen again. I recognised her father's voice on the news before I saw the pictures. We'd been friends at uni but had lost touch when I'd distanced myself in shame from all but my closest medic friends. For weeks, months, years afterwards, I followed the story. I wept for Madeleine's parents. I saw how destroyed they were, and yet how they kept going. And I was appalled at my own weakness after a loss that didn't measure against their tragedy. Appalled and ashamed. I couldn't even write to say how sorry I was.

I told Evelyn I was planning to go back to work full time. 'I'm not sure that it is a good idea,' she said. 'I think you are still too fragile.'

'I have to,' I said. I was crying, as usual. I needed papers for the research assessment exercise. I was in the middle of a set of experiments that required loads of after-hours if I was going to get the results in time. A big group from another institution was threatening to muscle in on my project. I was really going to have to go at it to make sure I came out on top. My boss wanted me back. He'd fallen for the charade. After all the support he had given me, I absolutely couldn't let him down. 'Fuck,' I said. 'Fuck.'

Evelyn handed me a tissue.

I took it from her and twisted it between my fingers. 'I'm not sure I can do it any more.'

The enormity of what I'd said sat between us for a while. Without my work, I was nothing.

'If you hadn't been a doctor or a scientist,' Evelyn asked after a while, 'what would you have done?'

I didn't answer. I felt foolish.

'Go on,' she said. 'What else did you want to do?'

'I wanted to be a writer.'

My English teacher at secondary school had a Glaswegian accent calloused by cigarettes and alcohol. In rasping tones, she would alternately illuminate Shakespeare for us or take the piss when we didn't get it. She was a genius in reverse psychology, getting even the diehard clowns in the class to actually do some work. She was the first person to champion my writing. The only time she ever lost it with me for real was when I told her I wasn't doing sixth-year studies English, and I wasn't going to do English lit at uni.

'Why do all the clever ones think they have to do medicine?' she said. 'You should write. It's a waste.' The weight of her disappointment didn't particularly affect me. I was seventeen and I knew better.

Her words came back to me now. Maybe I could be a writer. Maybe I could pick up where I had left off all that time ago. But there was no evidence to suggest that I still had it in me. Quite the opposite. I hadn't written anything for years other than letters to friends, dodgy poems in my more tortured periods, and scientific papers that were hardly great works of literature. The most recent stuff was the journal that I'd kept in hospital. None of it was what you would call enjoyable reading.

What the hell was I thinking? I was a research scientist. I had a job. A career. Writing wasn't a career. It was a dream. A delusion. A stupid fucking idea. And I was a stupid fucking idiot even to think it.

66

I was starting to unravel. It felt physical. Exposed. As if I could pull a tab in my head and it would unwind and fizz like the insides of the golf balls we used to find on the dunes and unpeel when we were kids. The Australia conference was approaching. It would be the first conference since I'd been in hospital. Everyone there would know. Or maybe they wouldn't and I'd have to pretend and find some crappy explanation for my long absence. There would be rival groups there who would think nothing of tearing my work to shreds. Of tearing me to shreds. There would be too much beer and I'd stand out because my beer-drinking skills were diminished. I wouldn't recognise people I knew. My laugh would be too harsh, too fake, and everyone would see through me. I would almost certainly cry in public. I would definitely embarrass myself. The more I thought about it, the more the whole thing terrified me. My anxiety-sweating cranked up to an all-time high. My tremor was back – nothing to do with the drugs this time – and it had begun to affect my lab work. My gels were a mess because I couldn't pipette the tiny volumes into the wells without it leaking out everywhere. When I tried to weigh out microquantities of chemicals, the spatula shook and sprinkled the balance with chemical dust. Measuring cylinders and beakers got smashed in the sink, victims of my agitation. I dropped flasks of bacterial cultures. Spilled precious reagents. Misread protocols. I wanted to pull that tab in my head. I wanted to unpeel, unwind. I wanted the relief of not having to try to hold it together. I wanted to drink the fucking poison.

A few days after my conversation with Evelyn, I dropped in on the department administrator to collect travel-insurance documents for the conference. Usually, I would stay for a chat, but that day I wanted to get out of there as quickly as possible. I was hyped and on edge. I didn't want to have to fake how happy I was to be going to Australia.

'Are you OK, Helen?' she said, handing me the documents. 'You look terrible.'

Fine, I wanted to say, *I'm fine*. But the words snagged in my throat. Tears were pooling, colluding to betray me. I tried my hardest not to blink. I was terrified to cry in front of her. Terrified of what it might precipitate.

'Come on,' she said. 'Let's go for a coffee.'

In the staff café in old Gilmorehill, I sat opposite her and stirred imaginary sugar into my black coffee. The clink of the spoon against the cheap crockery was muffled by the dark wood panels and heavily curtained windows. This was a hallowed place, out of bounds when I had been a student, and beneath my present despair, I felt a wistful glow of pride at being permitted to be there. In tones that matched the fading carpet, I told her what was going on. Told her how close I was to unravelling.

'I've got two choices,' I said, sniffing back tears and pretending to joke. 'I can either kill myself or move to France and be a writer.' It wasn't until I said it out loud that I realised how the plan had been coalescing in my mind. Mark worked for a company that had an office in France. Maybe we could move. Maybe I could reinvent myself again. Only this time, under the sun. There was only the small detail that I hadn't mentioned any of it to Mark.

'Well, that's not exactly a hard decision to make,' she said. 'Can I come with you?' We finished our coffees and she walked me back down the hill to the research institute and into the building, but she wouldn't let me back in the lab. She stayed with me while I collected my things. Then she phoned Mark to come and fetch me, and escorted me off the premises. She didn't want a suicide on her hands.

Leaving was both a relief and a catastrophe. I had gone backwards. Plummeted downwards at a startling pace. I cried. I was inconsolable. Desperate. I couldn't see a way out. If I gave up work, I'd be a nobody. But if I didn't, I faced the prospect of a life of crippling anxiety, of crises, of soul-destroying depression. And of the very real chance that one day I'd kill myself. Which wasn't really compatible with the job either.

Within a day I was back in Ferguson House in turmoil. The ward had moved to a new building with single rooms and individual bathrooms. That wasn't the only change. I was completely out of the way of being a patient. I couldn't fit back into the rhythm of the ward at all. I tried doing jigsaws and listening to the radio but my thoughts refused to settle. I talked to Mark about France and he spoke to his company. We came to a decision.

'I think I'm going to give up work,' I told Dr Lorimer when he came on his rounds.

'At last,' he said, his hair standing on end. Although instead of its usual panic, this time it was with delight. For years, he had wanted me to consider this option. It was an option I had so strongly resisted that he had given up hope of me ever accepting it. I felt a little shamefaced at how long it had taken me to come to terms with my own limitations.

I told John Lamb the same thing. I said I wanted to write a book. If I couldn't make a difference with my research, I wanted to make a difference with my writing. As I told him, I felt an obligation to use the brains that I was born with. Instead of calling me out for my conceit and my delusions of grandeur, he smiled. 'Go and make a difference,' he said. 'Go and write that book.'

I had been seeking, and I had received, permission.

Whenever we make the trip back to Glasgow, I avert my eyes when I pass the research institute. It is with shame and regret and a touch of longing, the same way I can't watch *24 Hours in A&E* on the TV and see the doctors who stuck at it, who kept going through the hideous working hours, the emotional trauma, the lack of family time, the all-consuming pressure of the job and the postgrad exams and further training. It forces me to face what I could have done if I had been able to tough it out. But I couldn't. I have to accept that. Whatever the whys and wherefores, the explanations or excuses.

The hospital where I was in ICU has been demolished now. I passed the wreckage recently and a shadow flitted over my grave. I wasn't sure if I was pleased or sad that the building had gone. Its presence could no longer bruise my heart but the ghost of who I was is still there, restless in the ether.

France

Addendum

No one knows the true meaning of love until they have a child of their own. It changes you for ever, makes you re-evaluate your life, makes you so protective you would die for them. Or so I have heard innumerable times. It makes me furious. My heart bursts with love for my nieces and nephews and I would lay down my life for them. I don't want to hear that it isn't real love. But maybe it is true. Maybe love for your own child is different. I'll never know for sure.

When you've lived most of your adult life with suicidal ideation, the first grey hair comes as a bit of a shock. I pulled it out, of course, but I guess that strategy is time-limited. Given everything that has happened, I should look in the mirror and rejoice at the signs of ageing, the slight sag of the skin at the angle of my jaw, the fine lines around my eyes and sun spots on my cheeks, a squinty tooth that daily becomes more squinty and makes me look like my dad. I never expected to make it past forty.

It took years before I could confidently say that I was well. I still take daily antidepressants and, on the days when I feel echoes of the stress and anxiety that are hideously familiar, I have to remind myself that they are just that – echoes – and do not herald a relapse.

These days I'm better at accepting my limitations. Better at managing my memory problems and the after-effects of what happened to me and to my brain. As a writer, it's embarrassing that I can't remember the plot of the novels I have read but instead am left only with an emotional memory of the books. Memory loss and the tricks that time plays on me can lead to awkward situations, but it is easier to be open about it than to pretend otherwise. And I still feel guilty about my easy life but at least now I appreciate the joy of it. I'm still waiting for the shock, though. Still expecting it to hit me. That bomb blast that will shake me to my core when I fully comprehend what might have happened.

In France, we rented an apartment near a forest, close to a river. Bureaucracy and the vagaries of the French postal service aside, the first few months were heavenly. Unfamiliar sunshine, warm autumnal days, sea swimming in September. Perched villages, alpine walks, fruit and flower markets. Mark went to work and I read and worked on my French and kept up my fitness with long runs along the edge of the river, skipping over stepping stones, past lizards warming themselves in the sun, and dodging the scratch hollows in the mud made by the wild boar.

Every day was a doddle. I should have been thriving. But before long, my mood began to founder. I had no work to justify my existence. No children to justify my lack of work. I didn't know who I was any more. Once again, I found myself trapped inside a loop of depression and self-recrimination. There was a sad inevitability to it all. As one of my friends had warned me before we left, the blue sky didn't necessarily make everything right.

Early on I was referred to a psychiatrist, a Danish woman who thankfully spoke to me in English. The first thing she told me was that she didn't have any beds of her own in any of the wards, that the hospitals here were old-fashioned and treatment outdated, and I should therefore do my best to stay out of them. Oh, and how was my French?

'Basic,' I said, bemused by the idea that she thought it would be within my control to decide whether or not I would ever have a hospital admission.

'Well, you must ensure that you are prepared,' she said. 'You must quickly learn to say, *I am depressed and I want to kill myself.*'

I laughed but she wasn't joking.

Later, when the subject of children came up, she scoffed and said they were overrated.

'Get a dog,' she said.

I stopped seeing her soon after.

While I wrote and dossed about, Mark worked and worked and carried on. He never complained. French lessons and gym classes provided some external shape to my life. I worked as a volunteer and did the odd bit of teaching. As time went on I met new friends. Thanks to John Lamb and Evelyn, I had answers. Literally. They had given me the lines to answer the hard questions and the capability to give the full explanation if it was ever required.

'Not any more. I stopped work because I was unwell.'

'Children? Sadly, no.'

'Just me and my husband and the cat.'

'A proud auntie.'

★

It was writing that kept the nightmares at bay. The ones where I'd hammer down the door of my ex-boss and beg him to take me back.

I wrote poetry and short stories. I did courses. I passed exams.

I wrote a novel which had filled my head for years. If I can attribute my recovery to one external factor outside of the support that I had from the people closest to me, I would say it was writing that novel. Writing wasn't therapy per se. The novel is not like this book. It is not autobiographical in any way, except perhaps accidentally. But the characters kept my thoughts occupied while slowly but surely my soul healed in the background.

These days I am overwhelmingly thankful that I didn't die that night. There is so much I would have missed. The infinite joy, the laughter, the tears, the privilege of a life shared with Mark, with my family, with friends, and with the kids, related and unrelated, who make my heart sing. And the private moments that nourish the spirit. The flash of a kingfisher at the river bank. The shadows of an olive grove. A wild orchid clinging to a mountainside.

Over the years I've thought a lot about suicide, about those who complete and those who survive, and those who are left piecing their lives together in the aftermath. The tragedy of it turns me inside out. I think too about beloved friends lost too early to illness and accidents, and I think about their loved ones and how in their shoes, I might be angry with or resentful of someone like me, so reckless with their own life. And I marvel at how astonishing and how forgiving people are. Because however much I try to show myself the compassion that I would show a stranger, I find it hard to forgive myself.

I often think about what would have happened if I had died that night. How it would have affected Mark and my family and friends. Of how awful and unjust it would have been if he or they had had to suffer blame or guilt that they hadn't done enough to keep me safe. Because they did everything and more.

I've thought a lot, too, about my reasons for writing this book. I am torn between believing that sharing experiences like this helps lift the stigma of mental ill health and worrying about the consequences of sharing – for myself and for anyone who might read it. I remember when I was at my most ill, how unhelpful it was, damaging even, when people assured me that things would get better. How could they know? How could they possibly know? Promises based on thin air were too easy for me to disregard. And yet, and yet . . .

I hope that no one who reads this has ever found, or will ever find, themselves being dragged under by the force of their depression. But if that is you, if you are frantically treading water to stop yourself drowning and the moment comes where you think you can't do it any more, the moment when you want to give in and let the sea take you, I beg you to keep going. You have endured so much. I implore you to endure just a few minutes, a few hours, a day more. And please, please, call out for help. The help when it comes might not steer you to dry land but it might be the lifejacket that lets you turn on your back and float, the thing that lets you rest awhile, that keeps you afloat a little bit longer. Survival isn't always about kicking against the waves. Tomorrow the tide might turn and wash you ashore.

★

John Lamb once told me that, when it came down to it, the only thing that counted in life was love. When the essay which formed the starting point for this book was published, one of my closest friends read it at work. She laughed and cried. Her colleagues wanted to know what was wrong.

'This essay. It's hard to read,' she said. 'But it's OK because I know how it ends. Because I know it is a love story.'

Acknowledgements

First and foremost, my thanks go to all the supporters of this book. Without you, it wouldn't exist. Not only am I indebted to you for your pledges but also for your generosity of spirit, your words of encouragement and your patience.

The first time I dared to put down in writing any of the events that are covered in this memoir was in an essay for a creative writing module with the Open University. I was extraordinarily fortunate that it was read by Melissa Bailey, my tutor at the time. Melissa, your sensitive response to my essay and your ongoing support of my writing gave me the courage to share this story. I am privileged to have you as a friend.

Since then, a host of wonderful people have been involved in the realisation of this memoir and in buoying me up when I doubted myself (which was basically all the time). My thanks go to Arifa Akbar for publishing the initial essay and for her incredible reaction to it; to Claire Black for her detailed and thoughtful feedback – *love lay down* is a much better book because of it; to my first readers, Rachel Holden, Tabitha Mwangi, Ruth Taylor and Monique Wass for being gentle with me and for being generally amazing; to Aliya Gulamani, Suzanne Azzopardi, Imogen Denny and all the fantastic team at Unbound, past and present, who helped me through the crowdfunding and editorial process, and turned my manuscript into the beautiful book that you hold in your hands; a special mention for Fiona Lensvelt and John Mitchinson for their unwavering faith in the book, which helped quieten my doubts; and to Rachael Kerr, editor extraordinaire. Rachael, without your belief in the book, it would never have happened.

And finally, to Mark, who isn't Mark, and Mookie, who isn't with us any more, and to each and every one of you who saw me through those difficult times or was there when I came out the other side. You know who you are. I love you.

Unbound is the world's first crowdfunding publisher, established in 2011.

We believe that wonderful things can happen when you clear a path for people who share a passion. That's why we've built a platform that brings together readers and authors to crowdfund books they believe in – and give fresh ideas that don't fit the traditional mould the chance they deserve.

This book is in your hands because readers made it possible. Everyone who pledged their support is listed below. Join them by visiting unbound.com and supporting a book today.

Patrons

Catriona and David Birnie
Hugh Holden, Will Holden
Malcolm Main
Rebecca Staheli
Toby Taylor

Supporters

Clara M Abrahams
Margaret Adams
Gail Aldwin
Lulu Allison
Catherine Allsopp
Katie Almond
Angela Anderson
Ariel Anderssen
Kathy Appleby
Joelle Arnott
Sabra Attrill

Lisa Badger
Julie and Alan Bagwell
Melissa Bailey
Heather Bain
David Baker
Jon Baker
Timothy C. Baker
Zoe Ballantyne
Paola Urbina Barnes
Karen Barratt
Simon Barrett
Dave Barry
Pauline Beattie
Costanza Benedetti
Pearline Benjamin
Sandy Bennett-Haber
Phillip Bennett-Richards
Kate Birnie, Rachel Birnie, Erin Birnie
Claire Black
Tom Blackie and Henri Myers
Georgia Blair, Cassidy Blair
Mark Bowsher
Ana Torre Brändle
Karen Breaden
Stephanie Bretherton
Mark Bridge
Abbe Brown
Annemarie A Brown
Jeremy Brown
Brian Browne
Melanie Burch
Kimberly Burke
Rosemarie Buttery
Ruwani Callwood (nee Gunaratne)
Alison Cameron
Helen Carlile
Paul Carlin
Susan Carlin
Tim Cashmore
Liz Champion
Thalia Charles
Lisa Churchman
Sue Ciechanowicz
Robert Clafferty, Aileen Forsyth
Joni Clifford
Janie Collie
Eileen Corroon
Jeremy Coutinho
Alister Craig
Paul Crawford
Lesley Crerar
Marcus Cross
Heather Cueva
Eileen Cullen
Deirdre Cunningham
Tom Cunningham
Heather Cuny
Annette Danaher
Katrina Davies

Rick de Zeeuw
Hélène Delbouys
Imogen Denny
Veronica Josephine Dewan
Anne Dewar
Jackie Dewar
Emma Dhesi
Rachael Dickens
Christian Doerig
Jennifer Doig
Margaret Dolley
Lesley Donald
Laurie Donaldson
Eileen Donnelly
Hazel Douglas
Dena Doulaveris
Ailidh Dunn
Mark Earnshaw
Amira Abd El-Khalek
Sebastiaan Eldritch-Böersen
Katherine Ellis
Jennie Ensor
Gill Fenwick
Ranjit Fernandez
Jill Fisher
Mo Fisher
Molly Flatt
Naa Ardua Flohic
Jean Forbes
Kirsti Formoso
Darren Freeman
Rhys Fullerton
Geraldine Gallagher
Marie Gallagher
Morag Gallanagh
Dominique Gallard
Nicki Gallois
John Gardner
Laurie Garrison
Claire Gentil
Pauline Geoghegan
Tom Gillingwater
Gaije Gordon
Rita E. Gould
Munira Grainger
Karen Grant
Angie Greany
Posy Greany
Jo Greener
Martin Grocock
Julie Guihen
Peter Gumbel
Patricia Giangrande Hamila, Manuela Foley
Tansy Hammarton
Lesley Handley
Alison Harper
Toni Harper
Sarah Harris
Lisa & Andrew Hawkins
Rachel Hazelwood
Daxe Hehe
Anna Henrikson

Andy Herd
Jennie Higgs
Nikki Hirst
Rachel Holden
Roger Holden
Tony Holder
Daisy Homer
Jamie Houston
Claire Hugman
Jeanne Humber
Fiona Hutchings
Laura Hutchinson
Nevil Hutchinson
Donna Imlach
Jill Ingham
Dennis Jacobs
Chris James
Peter James
Christine Jarra
Deborah Jenkins
Sandra Johnson
Kerry Jones
Mary Jordan-Smith
Mary Jowitt
Heiko Kammerhoff
Graeme Kaney
Karen
Charlotta Kastensson, Vivien Schydlowsky
Tamsin Kavanagh
Mallika Kaviratne
DawnMarie Keay
Chelsea Kemp
Val Kemp
Christy & Shahid Khan
Shahida Khan
Gillian Kiely
Margaret Kinnear
Kirsty from The Boozy Book Club
Julia Kite
Sue Kyes
Brian Laundon, Monica Laundon
Sarah Ledingham
Catherine Lee
Fiona Lensvelt
Lieven Marita Levrau
Jennifer Lewis
Ching Li
Sofia Liebon
Clare Lipetz
Cathy Llewellyn
Keith Longworth
Brigitte Colleen Luckett
Anne M.Ardica
Alasdair MacKenzie
Fiona Mackenzie
Gladys Mackenzie
Heather Mackenzie
Lesley MacKenzie, Jan MacKenzie
Alison Macleod
Gillian MacLeod

Annette MacLeod, Michael Fotheringham
Jacqui Macnair
Kirsteen Main
Carolyn Mallon
Julie Mallon
Carrie Marshall
Jennifer Martin, Neil Gove
Tünde Mathe and Michael Clunnie
Grant Mathieson, Michael Hartley
Alison Maycock
Craig Maylor
Lauren McAteer
Pamela McCabe
Lynn McClean, Alastair Cunningham
Suzanne McClelland
Mark McColl
Annie McGrother
Elizabeth McIntosh
Jacqueline McKay
Myra McKinlay
Caroline McMicking
Karen McMillan
Taylor McNeil
Aidan McQuade
Jennie Elizabeth Mead
Julie Meikle
Leonarda Miglietta
Suzanne Milan
Gus and Jenny Mill
Naomi Miller
Luciana Bulhões Miranda
Linda Monckton
Dee Montague
Jenni Morris
Elaine Morrison
Alison Mottram
Rebecca Mulcahy
Orla Murphy
Barbara Murray
Cath Murray
Heather Murray
Jenni Murray
Tabitha Wanja Mwangi
Carlo Navato
Kathryn Naylor
John New
Jacqui Newberry
Chris Newsom and Jasmine Milton
Morgan Duna Nichs
Sally Norris
Conor O'Callaghan
Ros O'Sullivan
Caroline O'Connell
Martin O'Neill
Elaine O'Grady
Sola Ogun
Dr Justin Pachebat
Madeleine Park

Nastasya Parker
William James Parry
Maggie Parry-Mantel
Lucy Parton, William Parton
Lynda Paton
Helle Patterson
Nicola Sarah Pickstone
Sophie Pierce
Robert Pinches
Ian Plenderleith
Esme Podmore
Susan Pollock
Shona Potts
Victoria Powell
Ruth Prendergast
Laura Price
Vivien Price
Alison Priestley
Jude Pullman
Lorna Ramelin
Catherine Rees
Denis Rice
Fabien Richaud
Laura Richmond
Deb Roberts
Jude Roberts
Carol Robertson
Elizabeth Robertson
Lindsey Robertson
Harris and Max Rodger
Martin Ross
Alex Rowe
RuzaSova
Kerry S
Saj
Dana Sardet
Scots Whay Hae!
Karen Shaw
Gillian Shearer
Gordon Shepherd
Wendy Shepherd
Diana Sheridan
Jared Siess
Alison Sim
Claire Slade
Steven Smith
Susan Smith
Jane Spencer
Eugenia Sproul
Charlie Stark
Katie Stead
Amanda Stone
Jez Stone
Alan Strachan
Allison Strachan
Veronica Strasnick
Jeff Stratford
Malcolm Strath
Felicia Strehmel
Hulda Sveinsdottir
Catherine Taylor
Gabrielle Taylor
James Murray Taylor

Jo Taylor
Ruth Taylor
Scotty L Taylor
Sophie Taylor
Toby Taylor, Irene Taylor
Jane Temple
Russell Thom
Steve Thomas
Craig Thomson
Douglas Thorburn
Joanna Tindall
Sarah Tinsley
Tom
Malcolm Toms
Greg Trawinski
Natalie Trotter-King
Ann Tudor
Mel Turner
Dr V
Stephanie Vargas
Mark Vent
Valeria Vescina
E. K. Victor
Jo W
Angus Walker
Fiona Walker
Louise Ward
Neil Ward
Monique Wass
Amanda Watkins
Hannah Watkins
Lisa Watson, Lucia Delgadillo
Lesley Watt
Andrew Weatherhead
Miss Kate Webb
Sarah Webley
Jack Weeland
Alan Welch
Ruth West
Claire Westbrook-keir
Miranda Whiting
Katrina Whittingham
Diane Wilcock
Caroline Wood
Rowena Wood
Sarah Woolhouse
Alison Wright
Chris Yuill
Simon Yuill
Nilgin Yusuf
Stephanie Zia

A Note on the Author

Helen Murray Taylor is the author of the novel *The Backstreets of Purgatory* (Unbound, 2018). She was brought up in the Lake District and the north-east of Scotland. Before becoming a writer, she worked as a junior doctor in Glasgow and then as a research scientist in Oxford and London. The profound effects of a severe psychiatric illness, during which she was sectioned under the Mental Health Act, led her away from her intended career. Writing played a crucial role in her recovery. Her memoir, *love lay down beside me and we wept*, tells part of this story. She currently lives in France.

A Note on the Type

The text of this book is set in Bembo. Created by Monotype in 1928–1929, Bembo is a member of the old style of serif fonts that date back to 1465. Its regular, roman style is based on a design cut around 1495 by Francesco Griffo for Venetian printer Aldus Manutius, sometimes generically called the 'Aldine roman'. Bembo is named for Manutius's first publication with it, a small 1496 book by the poet and cleric Pietro Bembo. The italic is based on work by Giovanni Antonio Tagliente, a calligrapher who worked as a printer in the 1520s, after the time of Manutius and Griffo.

Monotype created Bembo during a period of renewed interest in the printing of the Italian Renaissance. It continues to enjoy popularity as an attractive, legible book typeface.